# STILL A MUM

*A story of modern grief and life after loss*

MEAGAN DONALDSON

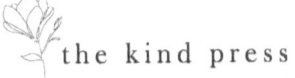

Copyright © 2021 Meagan Donaldson
First published by the kind press, 2021

All rights reserved. No part of this book may be reproduced, stored in a retrieval system or transmitted in any form or by any means, electronic, mechanical photocopying, recording, or otherwise, without written permission from the author and publisher.

This publication contains the opinions and ideas of its author. It is intended to provide helpful and informative material on the subjects addressed in the publication. While the publisher and author have used their best efforts in preparing this book, the material in this book is of the nature of general comment only. It is sold with the understanding that the author and publisher are not engaged in rendering advice or any other kind of personal professional service in the book. In the event that you use any of the information in this book for yourself, the author and the publisher assume no responsibility for your actions.

This is a work of nonfiction. The events are portrayed to the best of the author's memory. While all the stories in this book are true, some names and identifying details have been changed to protect the privacy of the people involved.

**Note to reader:** The book was written from when Violet Grace Donaldson was born, July 2019 to her first birthday, July 2020. When the author refers to the 'last twelve months' it is the twelve months since Violet's birth date.

Cover: Mila Book Covers
Internal design: Nicola Matthews, Nikki Jane Design
Edited by Georgia Jordan

Cataloguing-in-Publication entry is available from the National Library Australia.

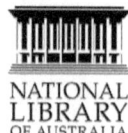
NATIONAL LIBRARY OF AUSTRALIA

ISBN: 978-0-6451392-1-1
ISBN: 978-0-6451392-2-8 (ebook)

*For my darling Violet*

*You will never be forgotten*

*Thank you for making me a mum*

*feathers appear when angels are near*

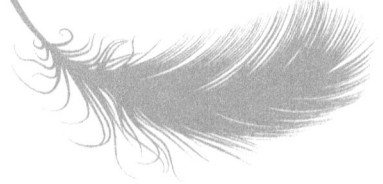

# Contents

*Prologue* The beginning of an ending — ix
*Introduction* The beginning — xi

| | | |
|---|---|---|
| Chapter One | Uncertainty and optimism | 1 |
| Chapter Two | The unimaginable decision | 15 |
| Chapter Three | A different kind of birth story | 29 |
| Chapter Four | Saying goodbye | 43 |
| Chapter Five | My good friend grief | 55 |
| Chapter Six | Say my baby's name | 69 |
| Chapter Seven | A different kind of trauma | 83 |
| Chapter Eight | Redefining me | 99 |
| Chapter Nine | A Grandparent's grief | 109 |
| Chapter Ten | Life in limbo | 121 |
| Chapter Eleven | Remembering Violet | 139 |
| Chapter Twelve | Why me, What next? | 159 |
| Chapter Thirteen | Everything I wish I knew | 167 |
| Chapter Fourteen | Still a Mum | 175 |
| Chapter Fifteen | Through Dad's eyes | 189 |
| Chapter Sixteen | Never forgotten | 199 |
| Bonus Chapter | Violet's impact | 211 |

*Pregnancy loss organisations and resources* — 225
*Acknowledgements* — 229
*About the author* — 231

## PROLOGUE
# The beginning of an ending

11 July 2019

To our family and friends,

It is with so much sadness and absolutely broken hearts that we share this news. At twenty-two weeks of pregnancy, after ten weeks of uncertainty—including extra scans, tests, an amniocentesis and an MRI—we received the news that our baby has an extremely rare and currently undiagnosable condition.

The evident symptoms and signs associated with our baby's condition are so rare that roughly only one baby per year in Australia is born with it.

We met with a range of specialists and were told the prognosis for our baby is poor, once born our baby would be likely to have a range of challenges, including and not limited to severe intellectual disability, respiratory issues, muscular problems, organ failure, seizures and an extremely poor quality of life.

Taking on board the information presented to us, we have

made the extremely difficult and heartbreaking decision to say goodbye to our very loved and very wanted, beautiful baby girl. This is not a decision we have made lightly and is something we know we will now live with for the rest of our lives. We find comfort in knowing that we have taken on our first role as parents by accepting all of the pain and suffering so that our baby doesn't have to.

Next week, I will have labour induced and we will welcome and farewell our beautiful baby, Violet Grace Donaldson.

We know that this is difficult to discuss and hear, however it is extremely important to us that our story is shared and doesn't remain a secret. There is no shame in what we have been through and what we are continuing to go through.

We know that this decision is only the beginning of an extremely difficult and challenging journey. We also know that silence is not going to help us learn, heal, or receive the support we need. xx

## INTRODUCTION
# The beginning

My story, like a lot of pregnancy stories, started out with a mixture of excitement and nerves.

At thirty years old, I had been asked more times than I could count when I was planning on having kids. For me, the questions started in my early twenties when friends, colleagues and well-meaning relatives began asking when I was planning on getting engaged to my long-term partner.

Once I ticked that box, the questions moved on to marriage then the topic of babies and children. (Friends have informed me that, even when you have a baby, you will swiftly be asked when you are going to have another! If you only have boys, you can be guaranteed you will be asked if you are going to try for a girl, and vice versa).

Despite many of my friends having babies, it wasn't really on my radar just yet. My husband and I had spoken about having kids for years, and it was something that we both knew we wanted. To be honest, he was ready long before me and eager to expand our family, but I just wasn't ready yet. I had other things I was focusing on and other things I wanted to do.

In conversations with my mum, I asked if I would *ever* feel ready.

It felt like such a strange concept; you go to bed one night content with your life and the next day wake up wanting a baby. I wasn't sure if I believed this shift would come and just kept on living my life as normal. I was fully aware of the monumental changes having a baby would bring and I wasn't ready to commit to that just yet.

And then, suddenly, I was.

I was ready.

*We* were ready.

This feeling everyone had spoken about had finally found me, and I was ready to expand our family.

Chris was elated and we agreed that we wouldn't tell anyone that we were trying. We would simply surprise them one day with the news that we were expecting.

We didn't get pregnant instantly but, when we did, the feeling of seeing a positive pregnancy test was completely overwhelming. It was something we had wanted, and our dream was now a reality.

We were excited, and in complete disbelief.

We hugged and kissed but didn't really know how to react. It felt completely surreal that it had finally happened, we were expecting a baby.

We spent two weeks planning the best way to announce the news to our families. Our baby was to be the first grandchild on both sides, so we knew there was going to be maximum levels of emotion and excitement.

Thanks to Pinterest and Etsy the delivery of our news didn't disappoint. For each of our parents, we created a little gift—a book for my mum and dad, and socks stuffed into one another for Chris's parents.

With each gift there was a card that read:

> My dad/mum loved it when you read/played sock footy with them when they were little. I can't wait for you to do it with me when I arrive in November.
> Love Baby Donaldson.

Our parents were the first people we told, it was truly one of the most emotional and happiest moments. We were giving them the gift of a grandchild.

We shared the news with our siblings and my nanna with cute scratchy cards purchased off Etsy. The cards had hearts and once scratched revealed the words: *Congratulations, you are going to be a ...*

Each time we shared our news, we were quite emotional and in continued disbelief that this was finally happening to us.

Like many others, we made the decision to abide by the twelve-week rule and not share our news with anyone except our immediate family. We wanted to wait to get into the 'safe zone' before sharing our news with everyone else.

Although the decision to share pregnancy news is entirely up to the parents, we felt the definite pressure from society to keep the news to ourselves until we reached the twelve-week milestone.

Thankfully, we did a terrible job of this and excitedly told the people closest to us. I am forever grateful that we couldn't keep our secret.

Sharing the news with our closest friends and family in those early days was the only time in our pregnancy journey that we got to experience the complete joy and happiness that comes with expecting a baby.

Shortly afterwards, we received the news that no expecting parent wants to hear, 'There are a couple of concerns with your baby.'

There is a reason I didn't start this book with that moment—because, to me, our story began long before it and continues long after it.

As I begin writing this book, seven months have passed since I saw those two lines on the pregnancy test.

It has been six months since Chris and I entered that warm, dark room for our eight-week scan; we were so relieved to see a strong heartbeat. An amazing moment. Our due date was confirmed, and we had an absolutely adorable picture to show people. After that, we began to relax a little, thinking that our baby was out of danger.

The hardest challenge of my first trimester was trying to hide the news and the morning sickness that occurred almost all day, every day. I absolutely hated hiding what was going on with my body and wanted to share our news with everyone. The amazing thing that I had seen happen to so many others was finally happening to us and I wanted them to know I was now going to be a part of the club. I would be able to contribute to their pregnancy conversations and share my birth story when the inevitable topic came up.

Although there is always a possibility that things might not turn out as originally planned, we didn't think that anything like that would happen to us. We never thought our journey to parenthood would be shared with others outside of family and friends, or that we would be writing a book. Our pregnancy felt so very normal. Everything that we'd hoped and dreamed about, everything that you see in the movies.

But our story didn't come with a fairytale ending.

As I write this, I am officially on maternity leave with no baby. Instead of planning my baby shower, I am finalising the details of my daughter's memorial.

We often find it difficult to believe that this is how things turned out. That feeling of disbelief we felt when we discovered we were pregnant was nothing compared to what happened five months later. The surreal feeling of expecting a baby was nothing compared to the moment we said goodbye to her.

This isn't only the story of our daughter, Violet.

It is a story about loss, life and love.

I began writing small parts of our story as soon as I arrived home from the hospital as I was terrified I would not remember the smaller details of Violet's life. One of my biggest fears throughout all of this has been that Violet will be forgotten and having our story recorded has helped me ensure that this will never be the case.

When you've lost a baby, the path you must travel is yours

alone. There is nothing anyone can do or say to take the pain away. No one can change what has happened and no one can bring your baby back. But by hearing stories from others who have walked that same path, it can help you feel less alone.

Over the next sixteen chapters, I wish for the words in these pages to help anyone who has experienced their own pregnancy loss to know that they are not alone. In sharing the details of our story, I hope to create space for others to have the courage to share theirs.

I am no expert in pregnancy loss, I am a Mum who has lived through the experience.

As I continue to share our story, I realise how much stigma and shame still exists surrounding pregnancy loss. Despite being common, it continues to be a taboo topic no one wants to talk about. We have also experienced the not-very-commonly-spoken-about taboo of the already-taboo topic of pregnancy loss, termination for medical reasons.

Throughout our heartbreak, grief and loss, I have learnt to find some joy in little things and have developed a renewed appreciation for life.

Some parts of this book are hard for me to read, but I've fought the urge to delete them. My mindset is very different now to when I wrote some of these chapters—that's all part of the journey of healing! Everything you are about to read was my truth at the time and, although my feelings about certain experiences and heartbreaking moments have shifted (because it turns out time does heal or at least alter your memories), I want to take you on my full experience.

If my words can help anyone on their journey or deepen someone's understanding of pregnancy loss, I will be incredibly happy—despite a year that fractured my heart, turned my world upside down and taught me more than I could ever have imagined before falling pregnant.

*When you've lost a baby, the path you must travel is yours alone. There is nothing anyone can do or say to take the pain away.*

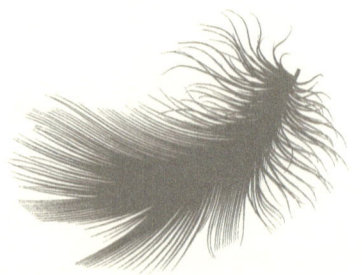

CHAPTER ONE

# Uncertainty and optimism

My husband, Chris, and I are both incredibly optimistic people. Our natural coping mechanism is to hope for the best.

As part of our jobs, we're almost trained to be optimistic. We have to be in order to do our work to the best of our ability. We always look for the positives of a situation—although we sometimes need to remind ourselves to do this as focusing on negatives can be the easier option—and it always makes us feel better to do so.

Instead of being annoyed that we accidently took a wrong turn on a drive somewhere, we like to refer to it as taking the scenic route. We prefer to think that grumpy shop assistant is a nice person and may be dealing with things we can't see. We didn't worry at all about it raining on our wedding day even though it was predicted—and it didn't!

So, throughout the time we were trying for a baby we remained optimistic that it would happen to us eventually. We have learnt that approaching life with a positive outlook influences our experiences and often the people we interact with. As clichéd as it sounds, we both have an understanding that 'it's not about the destination but the journey', and we don't ever want to spend our journey focusing on or expecting the worst.

We had told our close family and friends the date of our twelve-week scan. We told them that once we received the positive news, they were welcome to join us in shouting it from the rooftops: 'We're having a baby!'

Naively, we didn't actually consider the possibility that something could be wrong, or that we would be leaving the clinic with anything but excitement.

Isn't ignorance bliss—for a while!

We were one month off celebrating our one-year wedding anniversary when we excitedly found out we were expecting. Our baby was a very much wanted and not-so-subtly hoped for first grandchild on both sides. It had taken us seven months of hoping to expand our family before we received the life-changing news.

We had started our journey with the relaxed attitude that if it happens, it happens. After a few months, our relaxed attitude started to diminish as I wondered why it wasn't happening for us. We eventually decided to introduce ovulation sticks and then a few months later—with no pregnancy or baby in sight on recommendations—we turned to acupuncture, and both had weekly appointments complemented with disgusting muddy-water-tasting herbs.

Ever since we'd started trying for a family, nine years after we were introduced by friends, I had thought about the moment we'd see the life we created and know that in nine months we'd hold our baby.

Chris and I are both parental people and, through our jobs, spend every day with children. At first birthday parties and barbecues, we were always the ones playing with our friend's kids. I have played countless games of duck, duck, goose and been to more than my fair share of play centres.

Throughout our dating lives, Chris and I would often discuss how we would hope to raise a child. When we went on holidays, we would note the places that it would be good to come back to when we had children. We bought our house because it was a good size to raise our family and was close to good schools. Having a family was always part of our discussions and decisions.

The day I took the pregnancy test, I already had a strong feeling I was pregnant. I did the test in our ensuite. We sat together on the bed waiting the five minutes before we could look and see the result.

When we saw those two lines we were completely overjoyed. We couldn't believe we were finally going to be having a baby. We sat together in complete disbelief, hugging with tears in our eyes.

On the morning of our twelve-week scan, Chris and I drove separately because our plan was to return to work where we would share our news. We couldn't keep the pregnancy to ourselves any longer and were so excited for our colleagues to join in on our joy.

When my name was called, we entered the same room where

four weeks earlier we had seen our tiny baby for the first time. I laid on the bed as the sonographer let us listen to the heartbeat again.

'It sounds strong!' she said.

We looked at the various parts of our baby's body, and she continued to explain each body part as she moved on.

'We've got a cheeky baby here,' she said, as she began pushing at my stomach. Our baby wasn't behaving, she joked, and she couldn't see what she was looking for. She needed a second opinion.

It's a parent's worst fear. A sonographer saying they'll just need to leave the room to get a 'second opinion'. Worse still, there wasn't another doctor available so we were told it was best for us to go home, for now, and that a doctor would most likely get in touch with us.

This wasn't how it was meant to be.

The twelfth week of pregnancy is meant to be an important and exciting milestone. It marks the end of the first trimester. It's considered the 'safe zone' of pregnancy because the chances of miscarrying lessen. When you hit twelve weeks, you're meant to be in the clear. Or so all the books say.

For me, the twelve-week pregnancy scan was the beginning of our incredibly challenging journey. We never entered a safe zone when we reached that special milestone; instead, our ideas of parenthood were turned upside down, and our happy announcement evaporated when we saw the look on the specialist's face.

The twelve-week appointment was meant to be the end of

'the wait'. The end of the period of secrecy before you could share your news with the world. But for us it was only the start of a surreal period of waiting that went on for hours ... days ... months. A period of waiting that, in a way, continues even now.

You don't think it's going to happen to you ...

It was a Monday morning. I knew if I was able to focus that work would provide an excellent distraction from the reality of our situation. I never get any downtime at work so wouldn't have a chance to run through all the possible negative outcomes. With a bit of hope I could just block it out of my mind until I had more information.

So, I returned to work with a question mark over my head.

It might sound strange if you've never been in that situation, wouldn't you demand answers? But, at this point, they had no answers to give us.

Go home. Wait. We're not sure exactly what we're dealing with here. We'll schedule another scan when the doctor is available.

There was absolutely nothing I could do to speed up the process. Sometimes, not knowing means there is nothing to worry about. You can be as optimistic as you like, and there's comfort in that.

We hadn't received the positive reassurance we were hoping for, but we also hadn't been told that something was wrong. We left that appointment in a surreal state of nothingness, unable to comfort each other because we didn't know if we needed to, yet. All we could do was go back to work as we planned and somehow try to get through the rest of the day.

I went straight into a work meeting and sat in a conference room, barely listening to what was being discussed. A colleague, who knew about my pregnancy and my scan, excitedly peeked in through the glass door with an expression of anticipation. I pretended not to see her.

It's a strange and surreal place waiting to hear bad news or the confirmation of a heartbreaking diagnosis. Your mind wants to protect you by thinking of the best, or in some cases the worst. Is it best to hope for good news and risk being crushed by reality? Or, to decide that bad news is coming and rob yourself of that last hour or day of living in denial?

Would I have preferred to know what was ahead of us?

Déjà vu set in at our next appointment as the sonographer spent an agonising twenty minutes scanning my stomach, apologising for not being clearer with us that morning. Then came in the doctor who stared at the screen before uttering two sentences we'd hoped never to hear.

'Things don't look exactly as they should. Your baby has a couple of minor abnormalities.'

The type of person you are might impact how you react in that moment. You hang off the word 'abnormality' or you cling to the word 'minor'. Should we be heartbroken at the thought our baby isn't entirely healthy or hopeful that it could be worse and this is fixable?

The main concern with our baby was that there were two abnormalities, not one. One abnormality can occur randomly, but two abnormalities can often be an indication of some sort of disorder or syndrome. The head of our baby only measured two centimetres, so everything they were looking at was incredibly small. At this stage they couldn't tell us the impact the abnormalities would have on the development of our baby. We also didn't have enough information to determine if our baby did have a disorder or syndrome.

So, what was going to happen next?

We decided to go ahead with the pregnancy, even though we didn't know if we'd have a healthy baby at the end.

I wonder, now, if it would have been better to just find out everything on that day. To find out the true scale of what was ahead of us and have a looking glass that would allow us to see the day our baby was born.

Instead, we waited. Because, really, what other choice did we have?

In hindsight, the waiting made every decision and process more difficult. Making the decision at twelve weeks, while equally heartbreaking, would have been a very different process.

The plan moving forward was to firstly await the Harmony non-invasive prenatal test (Harmony NIPT) results. If they showed any risks or abnormalities, I was to return immediately to discuss a plan. If they presented low risk and with no concern, I would return at sixteen weeks for another ultrasound. This would allow our baby more time to grow and develop, which would provide the doctor and sonographer a clearer picture of what was going on.

We agreed to continue to keep the pregnancy to ourselves and had asked everyone who already knew not to say anything. Instead of excitement, our news was met with hugs of support and sympathy.

How would you cope with a wait that could end in heartbreak?

Over the next few months, we received good news. Our NIPT test came back low risk in all areas including Down syndrome.

At sixteen weeks, the cyst on the brain, the first abnormality, was still prominent but due to the size of our baby it still couldn't be determined how or if it would affect development. At the doctor's recommendation, we underwent an amniocentesis, a high risk and unpleasant procedure where they insert a ten-centimetre needle into your uterus to extract amniotic fluid.

More waiting followed.

At eighteen weeks, we were told the results of the amniocentesis all looked good. But there was still a long way to go.

With this news I was encouraged to continue to act under the assumption that my pregnancy would have a positive outcome. We attended the booking appointment at the hospital and were given a pregnancy goodie bag that I later threw in the bin on the day we arrived home from hospital without our baby. We booked in for our birthing classes and, although we didn't make any purchases, we continued to mentally prepare for the arrival of our baby in mid-November.

It felt like we were standing with one foot in two different worlds. So close to our dream of starting a family but also, at times, so far from it.

I looked pregnant. I had also begun to feel our baby moving

around at night when I laid on my back in bed, and I slowly began noticing it throughout the day too.

However, like all milestones in my pregnancy I was full of mixed and conflicting emotions. I knew that with every movement I was growing attached to a baby with a question mark over its head.

How would you cope in this situation?

How does anyone cope with an anxious shadow of uncertainty in their lives?

During 'the wait', as it would later be known, I began to implement tools and strategies to assist with my mental health in case the worst did happen. Every morning, I went out for a walk with my dogs before work and spent ten minutes cuddling with them on the couch, and practised a guided meditation followed by pancakes for breakfast. This went on for over ten weeks.

I was thankful for the cold winter weather, as I could create a uniform of layers of dark, loose clothing, scarves and jackets.

On a sunny day, I remember a lady at work looking at my outfit and asking if I was hot. I laughed it off and told her I wasn't whilst wondering if she could see the flush of colour on my neck and cheeks. Any opportunity I got I would rush back to the privacy of my office and take the layers off and cool myself down before putting my uniform back on and returning to face everyone.

I became a bit of a hermit on the weekends, exhausted after a week of pretending that things were okay, with no energy left to do anything. I didn't go to social events as I couldn't cover up in clothes like at work; if I wore regular clothes, people would know I was pregnant. I even had to make the decision to not attend one of my close friend's hen parties as there was no way I could hide it.

At our sixteen-week appointment, my doctor informed us that parents can make a decision to not continue with a pregnancy up until twenty-four weeks in Victoria. It was information we needed to know, but I didn't want to have to think about, yet. All I hoped for was not to be faced with that decision.

'It's not the result any of us hoped for,' she said

That afternoon I had a missed call from my doctor. We had an appointment booked in two days, so we just assumed she had positive news and didn't want to wait to tell us.

Nothing could have prepared us for that conversation. The beginning of a completely different ending to our story.

I can clearly remember everything about that phone call, as we sat on the end of our bed with the phone between us on loudspeaker. At twenty-two weeks pregnant, the MRI had clearly shown that the cyst was only a part of a much bigger issue. Our baby had an extremely severe and extremely rare brain malformation in addition to enlarged organs.

No surgery could fix it.

Neither of us cried when we were on the phone, it wasn't like the movies where people break down on the floor hysterically. Instead, we did our best to process the information and understand what the next steps were as we tried to find solace in facts and instructions.

Although from our twelve-week scan we knew it was a possibility, we never actually thought we would be faced with this reality.

Chris sat silently next to me as I paraphrased and repeated what our doctor had said to confirm I'd understood her meaning perfectly.

The conversation lasted five minutes and changed absolutely everything.

Up until then we had not Dr Googled anything, we knew the rabbit warren of anxiety that it could lead us down. Our doctor had told us the potential outcomes of our baby's brain malformation, polydactyl and enlarged organs. She had shared the syndromes they could be linked to and suggested we look them up to give us some more information.

Things were not okay.

The prognosis was bad.

'We're going to book you in with a geneticist to try to find out why this has happened so we can use that information for any future pregnancies,' the doctor said.

*Future pregnancies!*

My baby was still kicking and flipping inside of me, and the focus was moving to the next. Because it seemed that with this baby, we had no hope left.

Once we hung up the phone, we did completely break down. This was beyond our worst-case scenario. This was nothing we could have ever imagined.

In the immediate aftermath, Chris and I moved to separate areas of the house to start googling with the information we had.

Most of the time, when you google things, you can find some sliver of hope somewhere to hold on to. We couldn't!

Everything we read painted an even harsher picture. Once born our baby would be likely to have a range of challenges, including but not limited to severe intellectual disability, respiratory issues, muscular problems, organ failure, seizures, gross and fine motor issues and an extremely poor quality of life overall. That was if our baby survived the pregnancy and birth – even then, they would potentially have a short life span.

In my searches, I came across one article about a mother in the United Kingdom with a four-year-old child who had one of our baby's potential syndromes. She said on average she was in the hospital at least two to three times a week. Every morning she woke up unsure if her child was still alive. She talked about the pain her child experienced every day and how difficult it was to watch. She explained that through support groups she had met a couple of other children with the same syndrome but that they were no longer alive.

We had to decide.

To continue with our pregnancy or end our pregnancy, our baby's life.

This was by far the biggest decision either of us had ever been faced with. Up until that point our biggest decisions related to changing jobs or the location of our first home. We had never been faced with any decisions that were related to life and death.

When I was younger my mum had taught me to make a 'pros and cons' list for decisions, ensuring that the pros outweighed the cons. Unfortunately, everything felt like it fell into the cons category. There are not any real positives when faced with a decision like this.

I don't actually remember having a specific conversation about making a decision. With the facts in front of us we both just knew.

To this day, I am so thankful we were on the same page with this. We had a shared understanding about what this would mean for our child and for us as a family.

Although the information was damning, we decided to wait to see what the geneticist was officially able to tell us; unless they were able to offer us any form of hope in the way of surgeries or other options, we knew we were not going to be meeting our baby in November.

We knew we might never see our baby take their first breath or hear their first cry.

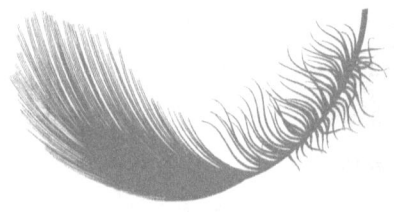

*Sometimes, not knowing means there is nothing to worry about. You can be as optimistic as you like and there's comfort in that.*

## CHAPTER TWO
# The unimaginable decision

In the midst of our heartbreak, we clung to ways we could be proactive. In between hysterical crying and apologies to the baby moving around in my belly, we needed to work out what was actually going to happen, practically.

For the next two days, we spent our time searching the depths of the internet and learning things that I wished I'd never have to know in my lifetime.

We decided to find out the gender of our baby which, until then, we had wanted to be surprised by. We spent a lot of time trying to find the perfect name as the ones on our list no longer felt right. We needed a name that had meaning. A name our baby didn't need to 'grow into'.

I was twenty-two weeks pregnant at this stage.

On social media and the news, abortion and termination were currently a huge topic of discussion. To much protest, America had recently made abortion illegal in multiple states. In Australia, there was also a law being debated in New South Wales. On a Facebook article, I read a comment that said anyone considering terminating a pregnancy after twenty weeks needed to 'get her head checked as there is something clearly wrong with her'.

There *was* something wrong with me.

My baby had no chance of a healthy life.

I couldn't believe that at twenty-two weeks of pregnancy, I was researching the termination laws in Australia. I had known that it was legal to terminate a pregnancy up until twenty-four weeks in Victoria due to it being mentioned at my sixteen-week ultrasound appointment, but until then I hadn't realised that it actually differs in every state in Australia.

If I had lived in any other state than in Victoria the decision wouldn't be mine and if I was over twenty-four weeks in Victoria the decision wouldn't be mine either. What would happen is I would have to submit the information to a medical board or multiple doctors who would make the decision for me. Whatever was decided was what I would have to do.

We knew we didn't have a lot of time.

Although the technical term for our decision is 'termination for medical reasons' (TFMR), and I have used that term since then, neither Chris nor I were comfortable using those words at the time. We felt and continue to feel that the word termination takes all the love out of our story and makes it sound overly clinical and simple.

Nothing about this decision was simple. When talking to anyone who isn't a medical professional, we prefer to say that we 'medically interrupted' our pregnancy or we 'induced labour early for medical reasons'.

Although it didn't require a lot of conversation, it wasn't a decision we made lightly. How could you? How do you even begin to come to a decision like that, or find the words to say it aloud.

In addition to finding out information about our baby's possible syndrome and brain abnormality, I spent a lot of time trying to find other women who had been faced with the same impossible decision. I read articles and went back to forums that had terrified me in the early stages of my pregnancy.

It was on one of those forums that I discovered the term termination for medical reasons. Once I knew that term and began to google it, a whole community of people opened up to me. When I typed it into Instagram, I found a lot of people who had been in our position. Stories you would never hear until you had a reason to search for that phrase.

I discovered that we were not alone. I devoured all of their stories, and spent hours taking screenshots of quotes they had posted that captured exactly how I was feeling. Quotes that read: *I carried you every second of your life and will love you every second of mine,* and *I would not undo your existence just to undo my pain.*

I read about their heartbreak and sometimes even slid into their DMs with the story of my own heartbreak. I have never been a huge social media user or even a big fan, but in these moments, I was unbelievably thankful to be able to connect so easily with people and feel just a little bit less alone.

I can't even imagine the pain and heartbreak of those before the internet. How incredibly isolating it must have been to not have the stories of others at your fingertips.

Through reading the stories of others and learning more and more about topics I wish I didn't need to know, I had even more questions and queries about what was actually going to happen.

The night before our next appointment, I remember lying in bed in the darkness as Chris slept next to me, drafting the message we planned to send to family and friends updating them on our story and what was happening. I knew that whatever the outcome, I didn't want us to feel shame. I wanted our story shared too if it made one parent feel less alone.

Our baby also deserved to have their story told.

During our decision-making period, from the doctor's initial phone call until our appointment two days later, we ignored all phone calls and messages. We had told our parents so they could be prepared but ignored everyone else despite countless messages from kind and caring friends. Each beautifully well-intentioned message felt like another stab to my heart as nothing about our situation was positive.

When we parked our car at the hospital, we didn't realise it would be five hours before we returned more broken than we arrived.

We made our way to the women's health unit and sat in a cramped space with three other pregnant women. At twenty-two weeks of pregnancy, I was so good at hiding it, I don't think anyone else realised I was carrying a baby.

We met another obstetrician who treated us with kindness and compassion. He asked what number baby this was for us and when I said it was our first his face completely dropped as he held my eyes and said how sorry he was. If I didn't already know how poor our prognosis was, his face would have given it away.

As I lay on the ultrasound bed once again, he asked us with all seriousness if we wanted to be told what he was looking at. I genuinely didn't know. Did I want to look at every feature of a baby that we were most likely going to be saying goodbye to? Or was it better not to see the little legs, the little arms, the face as we faced the reality of our lives together?

I could not stop crying as the doctor labelled all the parts of our baby. I held it together as best I could until the moment the sounds of a strong heartbeat filled the room, and I fell apart. I knew that this was, most likely, the last time I would ever get to hear that sound.

The obstetrician suggested we film it, so we did. In the months since then, I've caught Chris listening to it many times, each time with tear-stained cheeks and an obviously broken heart.

This was also the moment we discovered our baby's gender.

This was never how we imagined finding out. We had envisioned the excitement of being handed a baby in the delivery suite when the gender was announced. If not that, then the alternative in my mind was some sort of fun gender reveal. We could never have prepared ourselves to find out if we were having a boy or a girl whilst standing in a hospital room waiting to confirm the decision of whether or not we would choose to continue with our pregnancy.

In that moment we found out we were having a girl. All of our love and pain was amplified. This baby we had spent so much time discussing and hoping for now had an identity. Her name was Violet Grace and our love for her couldn't have been stronger. I felt so much more connected to her, right at a time when I was most likely going to say goodbye.

How do you say goodbye to someone you've never yet held?

We made our way from that appointment to the next with a box full of tissues in our hands, barely able to hold ourselves up. We were the people walking through the hospital that no one wanted to be. It was like a car crash; I could see everyone trying not to look at us, but they couldn't help it as our pain was so real and in their faces.

Our next appointment, in another hospital room ten minutes later, was with a geneticist and genetic counsellor who began by asking us what we knew about Violet's condition. Their job was to help us understand our options and to decide what was next. Although I think we already knew.

For weeks afterwards, I regretted giving them so much information. I felt we had made their job easy, as they just confirmed our understanding of what was going on with Violet. They reaffirmed what we had read in our internet searches and confirmed how severe the prognosis was. We were given a brochure called *Making a Difficult Decision: A booklet for parents who have received a diagnosis of an abnormality in their unborn baby*. At the conclusion of our appointment, we were told that there is no right or wrong choice to make.

It was entirely up to us, we would be supported either way.

Life or death.

One of our first questions was why all of our test results had kept coming back low risk. That low-risk result was what we had clung to and what had helped us keep going. It was so hard for us to understand how they could tell us that things were so horribly bad with our baby, but the NIPT test and amniocentesis hadn't supported this.

He explained it all to us using Google Maps as an analogy. The NIPT looks at the major chromosomal abnormalities, like the states in Australia, and our states were all good and didn't present any problems. The amniocentesis then looks at further chromosomal abnormalities, like the suburbs in Victoria, and our suburbs were fine as well. The problems our baby presented with were extremely rare and similar to the paint colour on the front door of someone's house.

There were no tests we could have done to tell us the information any earlier.

We left that appointment exhausted and overwhelmed with the magnitude of decisions we needed to make. It wasn't just one decision. There were many. Now and in the future. Pregnancy loss is a taboo topic with incredible stigma attached, and we knew that termination was the taboo within this.

I wanted someone to take the power of making the decision away from me. I was so desperate not to be the one to do it. I went through so many different thought processes, I wished I lived in a different state so the medical board could decide. I even desperately wished to have a late-term miscarriage.

I just didn't want to do it. I could never have imagined when I saw those two lines on the pregnancy test that this would be the outcome.

During the four hours we had already spent at the hospital,

our decision was clear. We had barely spoken about it. We just knew.

I remember walking back to meet our doctor and a lady asked if I was Meagan Donaldson. When I said yes, she placed a kind arm around my shoulders and said that our doctor would want to know what we had decided, had we come to a decision. Through gasps and tears I told her we had decided to end my pregnancy. I looked at Chris who nodded and agreed.

For the first time, we had officially said out loud that we had made the extremely difficult and heartbreaking decision to say goodbye to our very loved and very wanted, beautiful baby girl.

How much is good to know? If you were sick, would you want to know you were dying? If your child was ill, would you want their life to really lie in your hands? Or would you prefer to be in a peaceful haze of denial? I'm not sure there is a right answer to this question.

Something I really struggled with was that we had so much knowledge and understanding of what Violet's life would look like if we continued our pregnancy, and what our options were. Because of the type of people that Chris and I are, we did the research, and we came up with a plan. We were the ones, in the end, who suggested the outcome, who had to say the words first.

We made the doctors' and specialists' jobs easy. They didn't need to hold our hands and tell us that we needed to consider termination, we knew. They didn't need to tell us what a life with that level of disability would look like, we had an extremely thorough understanding. Although I knew no one could tell us what to do (oh, but how I wished they could!), I just wished that they had been the ones to deliver the information, not us. Chris did not share my doubts on this matter and felt that it was good we were informed, and the specialists just needed to confirm what we already knew. I just wanted something tangible to hold on to, to hear the words 'you need to consider termination' instead of us having to piece together the jigsaw.

My mum suggested I call my doctor and ask if she would have suggested it, if we hadn't. I chose not to call her, but instead drafted a text message. I wanted her response to be written down so I could read it over and over again for reassurance. And it helped a lot.

I also asked the doctor if we were really aware of our options. Had we missed anything at all? Her response was detailed and exactly what I needed to hear, as she informed me that termination is something always raised with patients when there are significant abnormalities.

If we hadn't said it first, they would have.

It's interesting to hear it from the expert's point of view. As a doctor, she informed me she gets an early idea of what the people she is seeing will consider and what they need spelt out. To her, it was clear we had a good understanding of our options. She thought we both knew, after the MRI result, that we only had one real option left, unfortunately.

She also wrote that she had no doubt this was the right decision for us and our baby, and then added that: 'If it's any consolation, the vast majority of people in your situation would make the same decision.' She supported us one hundred per cent in making it. She explained that we shouldn't second-guess ourselves and this was the most selfless decision we could make as parents. These were the exact words I needed to hear.

I saved a screenshot on my phone and sent it to Chris and my parents. If I had moments of doubt, I just reread those words.

To this day I have not second-guessed the decision we made, I am proud that we were able to take away our baby's pain and suffering. I just wish that this wasn't the outcome and that there were other options.

When I have shared an overview of our story with people who never knew I was pregnant, their first response has always been along the lines of *Why were you so far along in your pregnancy when that happened?* I completely understand this question and before my experience would have asked exactly the same thing. The scary truth is many abnormalities in babies aren't visible until the eighteen- to twenty-week scan because of the development and size of the baby. At twelve weeks a baby is only roughly the size of a lime and at twenty weeks a baby is roughly the size of a banana. There is a clear difference in size and visibility of what the doctors and sonographers can see.

Most people I have met, spoken to or read about who also made the excruciating decision to terminate their pregnancy for medical reasons actually didn't find out that there were any issues with their baby until the twenty-week scan. Each of them thought that they had a standard pregnancy with a healthy baby. They had shared their news with everyone and posted the cute social media announcement. Each of them began setting up nurseries and purchasing an array of baby items.

Although this is absolutely terrifying and scary to consider, it does happen and it is far more common than we realise, that is until it happens to you or someone you know.

It wasn't until a few months after Violet was born that I realised the grass isn't always greener. I was introduced to another mother by a friend of a friend who had made the same heartbreaking decision we had. But her experience, with her son Aston, was very different to ours in the delivery of her information.

In her thirties, Mary had what she thought was a relatively normal pregnancy. At sixteen weeks she held a gender reveal party with her closest friends and family and excitedly popped the balloon to discover she and her husband were expecting a boy. She painted the nursery and began making purchases in preparation for her baby's arrival.

Mary is a corporate lawyer, and this was her first child. She and her husband, an accountant, were the first in their friendship group to be expecting a baby and hadn't had much experience with children. They definitely didn't know any children with disabilities.

On the day of their twenty-week scan they ducked out of their workplaces between meetings to the ultrasound clinic for another glimpse of their beautiful baby boy.

Halfway through the appointment, the sonographer called a doctor to come into the room. It wasn't until the doctor took Mary's hand and looked her in the eyes and said, 'Your baby is incredibly sick,' that their world completely changed.

This is where our story differs.

Mary was taken into a small room with her husband, and the doctor told them they needed to consider terminating the pregnancy. When he went on to talk about the impact the various abnormalities and birth defects would have on her baby boy's quality of life, Mary told him to stop as she had heard enough. The doctor said he couldn't stop until they had a clear image of what their baby's future would look like once born.

Afterwards, they went straight to their GP, who called the hospital to book them in for the medical interruption of their pregnancy.

That morning they had been looking forward to seeing their baby and now they were discussing ending their very wanted pregnancy.

In addition to the heartbreak of making the decision, to ensure that baby Aston wouldn't suffer, Mary and her husband had incredible guilt for many months that they had such little knowledge and understanding of everything.

When we shared our stories, I couldn't imagine the pain and heartbreak Mary and her husband felt being bombarded with so much information in so little time; how incredibly difficult it would have been returning to a complete nursery, when all along you'd thought that everything was okay.

In turn, Mary told me she also couldn't imagine how traumatic it was for us to live with uncertainty for ten weeks.

Sharing our stories made me realise that there really is no good way to be delivered the information that your baby is not well or going to have a poor quality of life. Or to make a decision you never expected to make about a child you thought you'd see grow into an adult.

When it comes to decisions like these, there is no right or wrong.

It is incredibly difficult either way.

And, you have to take some comfort in that.

*How do you say goodbye to someone you've never yet held?*

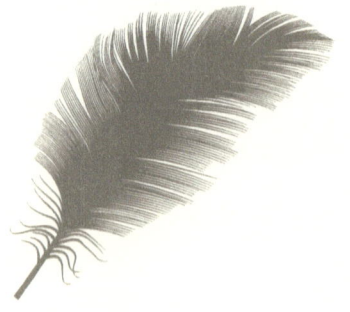

## CHAPTER THREE
# A different kind of birth story

I woke up early and stood in the kitchen as the morning light changed and rain hit the windows. This was the day my pregnancy hormones were going to stop. This was the day my body was going to start preparing to go into labour.

Despite the love and support I had in my life, in that moment I felt incredibly alone. There is a difference between talking about something and the actual reality of it happening.

During the last week I had become comfortable with our story, but I was completely distraught knowing that today was the day that would start the process. In my mind I knew that this was the kindest and most loving thing we could do for our baby, but that didn't stop it from completely ripping apart my heart.

We arrived at the hospital and sat in the waiting room with five other pregnant women. I still recall a phone conversation a very pregnant woman in a striped dress had with her mum. She excitedly repeated all of the information given to her by the obstetrician and told her mum that everything looked perfect with her baby boy.

I sat there with tears in my eyes, holding on to Chris's hand, trying not to let my sadness show so that I didn't upset or concern the other women in the room. The fifteen minutes we spent sitting in that room felt like absolute torture. I couldn't concentrate on anything—even looking at my phone wasn't a distraction.

I didn't have the capacity to read a magazine and didn't want to cause myself anymore pain by people watching. I just sat staring at the rings on my fingers in complete disbelief that this was my life. The desire to get up and run away from everything was incredibly strong.

Eventually my name was called, and we were guided into the consulting room to officially begin the process of welcoming and farewelling our very wanted and very loved baby girl.

In the hospital room, I was annoyed that there were baby photos all over the wall. I whispered to Chris that I was going to draw moustaches all over them if we were left alone. (We were left alone but I chickened out and settled on a small scribble on the wall next to me—so badass!)

We sat in chairs opposite the doctor and, for the fourth time that week, we had to share our understanding of the results and what we were about to do. After the process was explained in detail to us, I signed the consent forms to terminate my pregnancy for medical reasons. I was given a script for one extremely expensive tablet that would stop my pregnancy hormones and prepare my body to be induced.

This was the beginning of the end.

The tablet was required to be taken at home that night between 6.00 pm and 8.00 pm. For the rest of the day I kept checking the time, dreading the moment when I would have to swallow it down.

I read the pamphlet that came in the box. In bold on the very first line it said, *Do not take if you wish to continue with your pregnancy.*

I hated having to be the one to swallow it. I didn't want to do it. Once I swallowed that tablet, I knew that there was no going back. The weight of what we were about to do felt like it rested entirely on my shoulders. Although Chris was supportive, he couldn't take it for me.

At 7.50 pm I stood in the kitchen with tears streaming down my face. I swallowed the tablet.

Although the tablet didn't actually end my pregnancy or slow down Violet's movements, it stopped my pregnancy hormones and prepared my body to be induced. In the forty-eight hours before returning to the hospital to be induced, we packed as many memories as we possibly could into our final moments together.

We took her to the movies to see *The Lion King* and bawled our eyes out in the darkness of the cinema. We placed huge headphones on my stomach and listened to different songs, determining what she liked based on how much she moved. She wasn't a fan of any of Chris's music and much to my disappointment didn't seem to enjoy Beyoncé either. We had a mini photo shoot of my bump as we didn't have any pictures.

I found comfort in reading picture books to her, and I think within a day she had probably become one of the most well-read babies in utero.

On the day I was induced, I had to call the hospital at 7.00

am to confirm that I was coming in. I was absolutely hysterical making that phone call and could barely get the words out when the phone was answered.

My first time entering a maternity ward for a baby of my own was heartbreaking. Due to timing and circumstance, we hadn't even attended a tour or class to know what to expect.

I had always imagined my arrival in the maternity ward would be like in the movies where we would excitedly rush to the hospital as the contractions got closer and we prepared to meet our bundle of joy. Instead, we both couldn't stop crying as we were guided straight into our birthing suite, past all of the other expecting couples who were there that day.

We were introduced to our kind and caring midwife, a social worker and more doctors, and signed more consent forms. There is a huge amount of paperwork involved in a medical termination and each time I put pen to paper it was a painful reminder of the situation we were in.

The process for the induction was explained and, for the first of many times that day, we were told to be prepared that our baby may or may not be born alive. If she entered into the world alive the doctors would not resuscitate. Another form to sign consenting to this.

Everyone's story of giving birth is incredibly unique and there is no exception for the stories that involve loss. Each person I have spoken to who has lost a baby through miscarriage, stillbirth or termination for medical reasons has had a completely different experience. Some hospital processes and policies are different, which can impact the experience.

Some doctors and midwives are less experienced and less comfortable in delivering a stillborn baby and that can also have a huge impact on the experience. Some families have different views and ways of dealing with their loss and that can also impact the experience.

Through a discussion with one of my doctors, I learned that some hospitals have one very specific policy relating to termination of pregnancy for medical reasons. As a part of their policy, they insert a needle into the stomach of the pregnant woman to stop the baby's heartbeat prior to delivery. This is meant to alleviate the trauma and stress for the family and hospital staff around the uncertainty of whether the baby will be born alive or not. This did not happen for us, and I honestly can't imagine the trauma and pain felt by the women who have experienced that.

As this was our first baby, we had no other birth experience to compare to. We just knew that we had a different kind of birth story. One that unfortunately wouldn't end with the cries of a newborn baby, words of congratulations or excited visits from friends.

I have heard so many different stories of labour and birth; how painful and difficult it is, how some women enjoy every minute of it. Some people opt for drugs and others choose to do it naturally. One of the most common sentiments that all mums share is that no matter how challenging or difficult it was for them, they found the strength to get through as they knew that it was only a short time before meeting their baby and having them placed into their arms.

That sentiment provided little comfort to me.

I didn't know how I was meant to feel or how I would possibly manage to give birth to our baby girl. I have had many people say to me that they don't know how I did it and the truth is, I didn't feel I had much of a choice. What else could I possibly do?

I had been lying on the bed for an hour when I asked Chris to turn all the inspirational quotes on the wall around: *I trust that my baby and I will be fine*, and *I trust in my ability to birth my baby*. I didn't want to lay there and stare at the words, I knew that my baby wasn't fine and that things weren't okay. I didn't need the colourful Pinterest reminders of the end result that we were going to face.

The process of the medical induction began at 11.00 am. For the next twelve hours my body went into shock, and I experienced severe cramps, vomiting and extreme shaking. At twenty-three weeks of pregnancy my body wasn't ready to go into labour. I was given heat packs and wrapped in warm blankets. I had been given something to assist with the nausea and a dose of morphine for temporary relief. Chris sat helplessly next to me and gave me sips of water as I threw my body around, trying to find a position that could bring me some comfort.

The time between 4.00 pm on the Thursday and 12.00 am on the Friday was a complete blur. Through all of the pain, I honestly can't remember much of my thought processes during this time. I just remember being determined to meet my baby girl.

The medication to induce me was administered every three hours, and the hospital policy only allowed for five doses to be administered in one twenty-four-hour period. I had envisioned being given one to two doses of the medication before I was in full labour. I desperately didn't want to get to the fifth dose as I knew that they would then have to give my body a significant rest before trying again.

After each dose, the cramping and side effects got significantly worse, but my body did not go into labour. Chris was keeping our families updated with messages as they anxiously waited at home. My mum has told me that she and my dad just sat on the couch for the entire day unable to do anything else, just waiting for the next update on what was happening with their daughter and granddaughter. I honestly can't imagine how difficult the wait was for everyone in our lives.

The fourth dose was administered at 11.00 pm. It had been twelve hours since the process began, my waters hadn't broken, I was only one centimetre dilated. I was devastated that I had been in so much pain and so sick, but nothing was progressing. I had been told by the midwife that often with this medication things can begin to progress extremely quickly once labour begins.

Then only an hour after the fourth dose, the cramps I had been experiencing changed. I started having what I knew were contractions. Although this was my first experience giving birth, I had watched enough episodes of *Grey's Anatomy* to know that I was now in labour.

We pressed the button for the midwife and informed her that I was pretty sure I was in labour. I was told the doctor would come back to see me soon.

After a few more expletives on my behalf and several more presses of the button, the midwife and doctor returned to do an examination. It was confirmed that I was in fact in labour and ten centimetres dilated.

For a reason I can't remember, the doctor left the room. I had also run out of water and my mouth was extremely dry, so at my request Chris left to refill the jug.

In the midst of a contraction the midwife went to leave the room but, with a look I can only imagine as absolute panic and desperation, I begged her not to leave me alone. She was busying herself sorting papers at the desk when I asked for confirmation that if I felt the need to push I could. She said that I should.

Just before 1.40 am, Violet Grace Donaldson began her entrance into the world, breech and entirely in the amniotic sac. The midwife turned and looked at me with extreme panic. She gave me strict orders not to do any more pushing as she hit the button next to my head. The light above the door to our room began flashing as people came rushing into the room, including my extremely worried husband.

I was just ready to meet my baby.

There was no cry to be heard from Violet and minimal sounds from the midwives and the doctor. There were no words of congratulations or comments about who she looked like. The only sounds that could be heard were me asking the doctor and midwives what was happening and Chris crying.

It was the longest moment in a very long day, when I knew Violet had arrived but I couldn't see her or hold her, as the midwives and doctor did what they had to do for the autopsy. In my heart, I knew she wasn't alive. I couldn't remember the last time I had felt her move but I needed confirmation.

'Is she alive?'

I was told that she wasn't.

Although I have no doubt I cried when she was handed to me, I don't remember feeling any sadness. All I remember was being completely overwhelmed with love. I had never loved anyone or anything as much as I loved her in that moment.

The feeling of having my beautiful baby placed in my arms was everything I could have ever hoped for. Although I knew she wasn't alive, in that moment, it didn't matter. She was my baby and to me she was absolutely perfect. It is extremely difficult for anyone who hasn't lived through the experience to imagine, and six months ago I would never have been able to understand either.

When I held Violet in my arms it gave me an incredible sense of peace and filled my heart with so much love. I felt so calm looking at her perfect features and face. I couldn't believe that we had created her. She was the cutest baby I had ever seen in my life.

Once Violet was born, Chris's reaction and mine couldn't have been more of a contrast.

I felt so at peace and calm, and Chris was an absolute mess.

The tears did not stop falling from his eyes. He apologised many times for not being able to hold it together and in turn I felt terrible for not feeling sad enough or crying.

We dressed Violet in the most perfect pink knitted dress and beanie my nanna had stayed up all hours of the night to create. Chris wrapped her in one of her precious knitted blankets, also from my nanna, and he became the swaddle master. No one could wrap her up like he could. We gave her two teddies, one that had belonged to Chris's mum, and one knitted by my mum. The midwives filled in her birth card and Chris helped take her handprints and footprints.

After a couple of hours of broken sleep, we were moved to our room in the maternity ward. I proudly pushed Violet in her cot down the halls of the hospital to our room. She looked absolutely gorgeous in her dress, I was beaming with pride as we walked.

During our time in hospital, we were incredibly lucky to have a Cuddle Cot, one of the many amazing inventions that one month earlier I had never heard of—it has a cooling system that allows families to spend time with their baby once they have passed away.

That morning we had invited our immediate families to come and meet Violet if they wanted to. My parents and sister were the first to arrive and I could hear their crying before they had even properly entered into the room. There were hugs, kisses and tears shared. Seeing our pain reflected in their faces was the first time since Violet's birth I realised how truly sad it was. This was not how they were meant to meet their first grandchild and niece.

Shortly after, Chris's family arrived in the same way. They all had turns of holding our beautiful girl and listened attentively to my labour story. Each of them later said that they had arrived at our hospital room incredibly sad and heartbroken and left with a sense of peace. This wasn't what any of us had envisioned, but everyone who visited was glad to have the opportunity to meet Violet. She left everyone with a sense of peace and calm that they hadn't previously felt.

We were fortunate enough to have an amazing photographer from a volunteer organisation called Heartfelt come and take photos to capture our precious only memories together. Our photographer was absolutely incredible, kind, compassionate and professional. He spent just under an hour with us and the next morning had emailed an edited gallery of 106 incredible photos that we will forever cherish.

Our plan was to spend one whole day with Violet and then go home on the Saturday, but things didn't go exactly as planned. Due to an admin error, we were informed that Violet was unable to be discharged from the hospital to go with the funeral director. As it was the weekend, the error was unable to be rectified until Monday. For about thirty minutes I was furious; we had mentally prepared to say goodbye on the Saturday and I had felt this was one more thing that was no longer in my control.

We were given the option of going home on the Saturday and for Violet to be taken to the mortuary until the error was sorted. I hated the idea of being ten minutes away at home and had visions of them taking my tiny baby to the mortuary and people not realising or forgetting that she was there.

This minor change in plans had completely shaken me, it was one more thing I hadn't expected and that hadn't gone as I had envisioned. It didn't take long for Chris to help me see the positives in the situation and suggested that maybe it was actually better than we could have planned. Maybe we were rushing home too soon, and now, although unplanned, we were going to get to spend a weekend together as a family.

After much discussion, that's exactly what we did. We had one beautiful weekend together with our daughter.

That weekend, Violet watched her first game of AFL lying on her dad's chest. I sang nursery rhymes to her and tried to take mental and digital photos of every inch of her body. I made sure I kissed every part of her and gave her all of my love.

In Australia, if a baby is born after twenty weeks or more into the pregnancy, they are given a birth certificate. I spent hours before being induced googling, trying to work out if my daughter would get one and I am so glad that she did. Having a birth certificate for Violet means that legally she will forever be recognised as our firstborn daughter. Her name will appear on her potential siblings' birth certificates and her memory will be continued.

If a late miscarriage occurs and a child is born before twenty weeks, then they don't receive a birth certificate. In some cases, a day can be the difference between having a birth certificate or not.

In one of the pregnancy loss Facebook groups I am a part

of, one mum shared her absolutely heartbreaking story of the loss of her baby boy. She experienced a miscarriage at nineteen weeks and five days, was immediately admitted into hospital and induced. She gave birth to her beautiful baby at nineteen weeks and six days. If her baby had been born four hours later, he would have received a birth certificate—but he didn't. As he was not legally recognised, her baby did not need paperwork to be discharged. She took her baby home with her and buried his body herself.

It is important for me to share Violet's birth story as there is an incredible lack of understanding surrounding pregnancy loss. Many people don't actually realise I experienced a full labour. One lady I know wondered why they didn't just do a caesarean and remove the baby. One of Chris's friends actually said he just thought the baby went away. I'm not sure where he thought thirty-one centimetres and 640g of baby just went away to!

Creating awareness of the birth and processes involved in experiencing pregnancy loss will hopefully help others have a bit more understanding of the grief that follows loss. Each pregnancy loss is unique and so is the journey that each family goes on.

All I can do is tell Violet's unique birth story.
A story that will never be forgotten.
And tell you what happened next …

*The feeling of having my beautiful baby placed in my arms was everything I could have ever hoped for.*

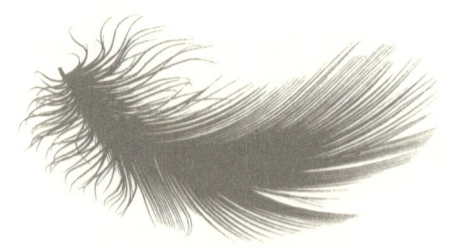

## CHAPTER FOUR
# Saying goodbye

Three weeks after giving birth, I sat on our couch at home and watched an episode of *Survivor* with our daughter nestled in my lap. I knew how strange it must have seemed to anyone but us. The television on, and an urn cradled in my lap. But I didn't want to put her down.

Six months ago, I would have thought, *That person is crazy.* I couldn't have imagined a world where I would be watching a reality television show holding an urn with my daughter's ashes in it.

But grief, it turns out, impacts everyone in different ways. And, although it can be healing to talk over and over a heartbreaking situation, there is also a time for distraction ... and a trashy television series.

Because there were memories I would do anything to avoid.

That morning, I'd woken up in hospital with our baby daughter—our final morning together.

I was crying. I slipped out of the hospital bed and picked up my beautiful daughter, trying to commit all of her precious features to memory. I could hear the distant echo of babies crying in other rooms on the ward, and my heart ached. I just couldn't see how I was going to get through that day. After all we had been through, I couldn't imagine how we were going to keep moving forward.

That was by far the worst day of them all.

This is also the most challenging chapter of the book to write, so far.

I still struggle to think about it without my heart aching.

Up until that moment, Violet was always with us. The day I took the tablet she was still moving around in my belly.

Everything we had been through had been leading up to this day and I wasn't ready. I wasn't ready to let go of her, and I didn't want to say goodbye. I was so thankful that we got to spend the weekend together as a family, but no amount of time would have ever been enough.

Now, our midwife let us know that the funeral director would arrive in forty-five minutes.

We had forty-five minutes left with our baby girl. How do you pack a lifetime of memories into less than an hour?

But I also knew that we couldn't stay any longer, as it wasn't fair to her or to us.

I had worked so hard to be optimistic and positive throughout my pregnancy, and I was terrified I would lose myself in the pain and not be able to function or move forward. I didn't feel like I had anything to look forward to anymore. Our whole future had been planned with Violet in it. But we had no choice but to say goodbye. Now.

'Letting go is an even bigger sign of love than begging for more when time won't allow.'

This is what our beautiful midwife said to me as she took my blood pressure that morning. I reminded myself of her words constantly throughout that day.

As we waited for the paperwork to be finalised, time felt like it stretched out for so long, but also like it was going too fast.

As we waited, I refused to let Violet leave our arms. We took one hundred more photos of her; we read to her, danced with her and sang to her. We kissed every inch of our girl and told her how much we loved her and thanked her for choosing us to be her parents.

I will never forget how much my heart broke with each minute that passed. It all felt so incredibly unfair as we changed Violet into her 'party outfit'. We decided we wanted to keep the clothes she had worn when we were together. So we dressed her in an Angel Gown that was gifted to us by the hospital, wrapped her in a rainbow blanket my nanna had made and placed a pink beanie on her head. We gave her a Bears of Hope bear that was gifted to us so that she wouldn't be alone.

And we sat in our chairs ... waiting.

We had already packed up our belongings and I had been discharged so we could leave the hospital as soon as Violet had. The funeral directors had provided us with options for our farewell and we had more difficult decisions to make, to leave Violet in the hospital room for the funeral directors to collect once we were gone, or to walk her to the car with the funeral directors and drive our separate ways, or have them collect her from the room.

To us, none of the options were positive as they all ended the same way—with Violet no longer being with us. In the end, we chose the last option.

Exactly on time, the funeral directors came into the room, introduced themselves and told us that they were going to take good care of our darling daughter. I could barely hear anything they were saying over the pain in my chest and tears in my eyes. I knew that she had to go with them, but I just didn't want to let her go. I just wanted to run away with her and never come back.

The funeral director placed a large black bag on the bed and kindly asked if I wanted him to place Violet in the bag, or if I wanted to do it. Chris and I gave our girl our final kisses before I placed her in the bag with her new teddy.

I have no idea how I had the strength, looking back.

The funeral director gently explained that, because he was taking Violet out into the public, he would need to cover her. We stood frozen in the room and watched as this lovely man—with so much kindness—covered our baby with a blanket and zipped the bag.

The funeral director shook Chris's hand and asked if it would be okay to give me a hug. The process took less than three minutes. In those three minutes my heart completely shattered and a piece of me left forever.

I have never in my life experienced physical or emotional pain like it. I don't think there are any words to describe the utter devastation of saying goodbye to your child. When I think back now it was almost like an out-of-body experience. I couldn't recognise the sounds in the room, they were completely primal, and they happened to be coming from me. We were completely helpless and there was nothing anyone could do to ease the pain.

We were joined in our crying by two of the midwives who had looked after us and Violet. They stood in the empty hospital room hugging and crying with us.

We didn't want to stay any longer than we had to and walked out of our room at the exact same time as another family taking home their baby. I could see the excitement and joy on their faces quickly change as they saw us and our obvious pain.

The contrast between the two couples couldn't have been more different. They were walking out with excitement and a capsule with their baby as Chris and I walked out with tears streaming down our faces and a bundle of paperwork.

We left the hospital with empty arms and broken hearts.

I can't explain the level of emptiness I felt that day and over the coming days and weeks. I was no longer pregnant, and I also didn't have my baby with me. My arms felt physically heavy by my sides and ached to hold our baby girl again.

How do you possibly go on from here?

We drove home in complete silence, both lost in our own painful thoughts. We hadn't been home in four days, so we were greeted with lots of licks and tail wags from our excited dogs.

The first thing we did was unpack our bags and water all of our plants. It sounds strange but it was so nice to do something completely mindless for ten minutes.

Our house was already filled with bunches of flowers and

more kept arriving by the day. I absolutely loved those flowers. They brightened up the house and were a reminder of how loved we all were. We received a plethora of cards too, outpourings of love and sympathy from friends and family. We even received cards from people we had barely spoken to or knew.

Our story was spreading, and everyone wanted to let us know we were in their thoughts.

I felt very quickly that not having my baby with me made it easier for everyone, including me, to forget I had actually given birth and gone through a full labour. The day after we returned from hospital, we went to the shops to get some photo frames to put Violet's photos in and I became incredibly sore. I had spent the last four days in hospital either laying down or sitting, the furthest I had walked was to the car.

I was angry at myself for going out so soon and for not resting and looking after my body. Now I had a painful reminder of labour that I couldn't ignore. But I also felt guilty laying around as I didn't have my baby with me.

When I was pregnant, all-day resting was acceptable and if I was feeding or nursing a baby it would have been completely understandable. But what category did I fit in now?

The mornings were the worst as most days I woke up feeling okay for a split second, and then I would remember what had happened and the wave of emotion would hit me. I cried on and off all day every day for the first few weeks. I could go a couple of hours without crying and then it would hit me again.

I spent so much time looking at Violet's pictures on my phone and even caught myself occasionally kissing the screen.

The first week at home was a complete blur and we did our absolute best to put one foot in front of the other.

How do you begin to form a new version of life, when your entire world is shattered? How do you look forward, when there is so much pain behind you and part of you doesn't want to move on—in case you forget?

We tried to establish some sort of routine that consisted of having a shower and making the bed each day (even if I hopped back into it!). Chris spent a lot of time on his computer watching videos to distract himself and I tried to be as busy as I could. Being busy meant I didn't have to think so I made myself a small list of tasks and worked through them.

I went online and printed Violet's photos, I registered her birth and tried to find any mundane task I could that helped connect me to her. I was also so terrified I would forget things, so I began writing down our story (part of which you're reading now!). I would sit on the bed each day with my laptop and bawl my eyes out as I recorded everything we had been through to that point.

I also spent a lot of time in the online community I had discovered when we had had to make our decision. I devoured each and every post and felt less alone reaching out and responding to others who had been through a similar experience.

We decided to write an announcement for our social media accounts accompanied with a picture of Violet's tiny hand holding my finger.

We wrote:

> On the 19th July 2019, our beautiful baby girl Violet Grace Donaldson entered the world still, but perfect. She spent only a moment in our arms but will forever be in our hearts. Thank you for choosing us to be your mum and dad, you have brought so much love into our lives.

For many people this would have come as a surprise as we had never had the opportunity to announce our pregnancy. Now that we had met Violet it was incredibly important for us to share her with the world.

I had a handful of people send me direct messages and I responded to each of them thanking them for reaching out and for their kind words. I also attached the original letter we sent to everyone explaining our full story. It was important to me that there was no shame in what we had been through and continued to go through and I wanted people to see that.

Another important task we had to do in those first two weeks was meet with the funeral director. It was another part of losing a baby I had no idea about. When we left the hospital, I hadn't realised that we would need to meet with them again to discuss the future arrangements. It obviously made sense, I just wasn't thinking clearly, everything felt incredibly surreal.

At the funeral parlour, I remember there being a mark on the wall of the room and I worried that we should have gone somewhere fancier. I only wanted the best for our baby girl.

We had choices to make, to bury Violet or have her cremated, have a formal funeral at the funeral home or do something on our own.

They let us know that even if we didn't have a funeral that they could place her in an angel coffin—which is the tiniest little coffin you could ever imagine, with wings on top—and we could sit with her and talk to her. We continued to be faced with more and more crappy decisions.

At this stage, neither of us could handle the idea of a formal funeral or memorial. The angel coffin tore my heart apart and I couldn't bear to think of her laying in it. We decided to organise our own private memorial once we were ready and to have our baby cremated.

I shakily signed the forms to formalise the process and was assured we would be updated by the funeral director when Violet returned to their care once the autopsy was complete.

Deciding to get Violet cremated meant we needed to find an urn. Instead of buying Bonds onesies in preparation for our baby we were searching in catalogues and online for the perfect urn.

Anyone who has ever had to type baby urns into a google search knows how truly horrendous they are and how difficult a search it is. The sadness of the task was quickly replaced by shock at how awful they were.

Discussing the tackiness of baby urns was one of the more humorous parts of the first parent support group we attended. One mum described them like shiny toys from the $2 shop with a Comic Sans font sticker on the top saying your baby's name.

One of the dads jokingly said some of them reminded him of his basketball trophies, but the basketball player was ripped off on top and replaced with a plastic angel. It's crazy what you find yourself laughing at in grief.

When sharing my story with someone I hadn't seen for a while, I would jokingly add in the part about those tacky urns, hoping it might lighten things up a bit. It didn't. I realised pretty quickly this type of humour was probably only reserved for those super close to me and anyone else who has lost a baby (obviously as long as their urn isn't a plastic figurine or trophy-like).

In online support groups, parents shared creative ways to store their baby's ashes, and I learned once again that you have no idea what you will actually do until you are in that situation. One mum had a bear made with her baby's ashes stored in it. At the time I couldn't think of anything worse.

We found a lovely lady who made Violet's urn out of pottery. She sent me picture updates as she made it, her kindness at this time made me love the urn even more.

We had discussed the possibility of spreading Violet's ashes at the beach. Chris also decided early on that he wanted to find a necklace that he could wear so she would always be with him.

Over the next few weeks, as Chris talked about the adventures he couldn't wait to have 'with' his little girl, I was incredibly jealous. So, I decided I needed to have some jewellery of my own so she could always be with me too and come on adventures. I also thought about the strength and courage I would feel having her so close, so ordered a beautiful violet-coloured ring with her ashes set in the stone.

I continue to wear the ring every day and at night place it next to Violet's photo when I go to bed. It is a beautiful reminder of her existence.

I'll never forget how tiny her urn was, the day Chris brought it home, with our precious baby who I had held in my arms inside. I was thankful that I had decided to get the easier-to-clean glazed urn option as standing in the driveway I couldn't help but smother my baby in kisses and tears.

We introduced Violet to our two dogs. Our female dog, Tilly, sniffed the urn and couldn't have cared less and our male dog, Charlie, just wanted to be near her. We had to pull him back to stop him from smothering her with too many licks. It warmed my heart to watch as it is probably exactly what he would have done if Violet were alive.

Although we had discussed spreading Violet's ashes in the ocean, bringing our baby home made me never want to be apart from her. Some nights she would sleepover in our room on one of our bedside tables, other nights she sat next to my computer as I worked on my writing. I also couldn't resist giving her the occasional kiss when I walked past.

We decided against spreading her ashes and kept her at home with us. Saying goodbye the first time was hard enough, and we are not yet ready or willing to do it again—any time soon.

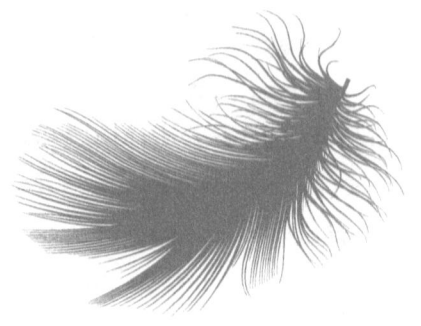

*Letting go is an even bigger sign of love than begging for more when time won't allow.*

## CHAPTER FIVE
# My good friend grief

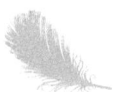

As Chris and I sat on uncomfortable chairs in a circle with six other sets of parents, I couldn't quite believe this was where we had ended up. It was the first night of our child and pregnancy loss support group—a group we had been sent information about through our hospital social worker.

It was six weeks since Violet's death and I was looking forward to being around other people who had experienced the loss of a baby or child. I was looking forward to sharing our story with others who could relate and understand how I felt.

When we arrived in the room it felt like a clichéd movie with crappy cups of coffee in the corner and awkward fold-out chairs placed in the middle. I was waiting for someone to say, *Hi, my name is … and it's been six weeks since my last drink*. One of the positives we noticed was the facilitator had violet-coloured streaks in her hair, something that before Violet was born wouldn't have been my cup of tea but now made me instantly like her.

The facilitator started the meeting by saying that there is no hierarchy of loss or grief. Everyone has a right to feel what they feel. And, as we listened to other parents' experiences and reactions to grief, I realised how true this is.

Each of the parents who were there had a completely different and heartbreaking story. One couple lost their baby at thirty-five weeks, the mum hadn't felt much movement and went to the hospital to be told that there was no heartbeat. Another mum had gone into premature labour at twenty-three weeks and despite the hospital doing everything they could to keep her baby alive and safe, she had lost him a week later. Another mum was there after experiencing what is referred to as a late-term miscarriage at sixteen weeks.

Not only were the stories and experiences all different, the reactions to grief were too. More than one person in the group mentioned that they wished they had died when their baby had died. Many people had mentioned that they had stopped sleeping and couldn't function during the day. Some people admitted to drinking too much and others shared that they were barely eating.

I once read in a book that everyone feels that their grief and loss is the most traumatic and none of them are wrong, because it is most traumatic to them.

Unfortunately, I found out there is no guaranteed step-by-step program or how-to handbook on getting through grief. I also found that the only people who are truly able to understand how I felt are those who have walked the same path.

*Grief is the form love takes when someone dies*—this is one of my favourite sayings I have come across since giving birth to our daughter.

All the knowledge in the world and all the preparation you do still won't prepare you for how it actually feels to lose a loved one. Or that is what I discovered after losing our baby.

From so early in our pregnancy, there was always the possibility that this might be our story, but that didn't make me feel any more prepared when the ending came.

I had never experienced life-shattering grief before, and I didn't realise how difficult it would be. I also didn't realise how uncomfortable it would make me, or how uncomfortable it would make the people around us.

Nobody really wants to hear about other people's grief—this is what I quickly found out.

It turns out, grief makes people extremely sad, even if you haven't had a relationship with the person who died. Perhaps it's because it gives everyone a glimpse into what can happen in life—what *will* happen to all of us.

In my experience, I've found that grieving the loss of an unborn child makes people even more uncomfortable. For many people it seems terrifying and all too real—to know what we have been through can happen to anyone without warning. For others, there is so much confusion and lack of understanding. How do you grieve a child you never got to meet alive? How do you grieve a child that only your immediate family got to meet?

I was hoping in going to the support group that we would meet other couples or people who had experienced the loss of a baby and maybe even make friends. Although I have been fortunate enough to be incredibly supported by friends and family, no one really understands how it feels.

I also thought it might be helpful for Chris to have the

opportunity to be around other men who had experienced loss. I had immersed myself in online forums and Facebook pages, and was regularly seeing a psychologist, but Chris was grieving alone. He spoke to me and the very occasional friend and that was it.

After the first support group, Chris mentioned to me that listening to the other men had been good, but what impacted him the most was the women who were there on their own as their husbands/partners wouldn't attend. He said listening to those women made him realise how important it was to support me and work through this as a team.

We attended the group only three times and each time tried to focus on it being a date night and a nice opportunity to talk about Violet. As our lives moved forward there felt like less opportunity to discuss her, so the support group offered us that chance.

Everyone at the support group was kind and supportive, but we didn't make friends. I'm not sure if it would have been different if we had attended more regularly, I don't think so. Despite everyone having experienced baby loss, no one could quite relate to our story.

The women who sat in the circle crying said they felt it was their fault their baby died and that they wished they had done something differently. Everyone else immediately consoled them and let them know that there was nothing they could have done to change the outcome. This wasn't the case for us, in a way I *was* responsible for the loss of Violet, and I could have changed the outcome.

Although there is no one-size-fits-all guide when it comes to grief, it is beneficial to talk and share your experiences. Because, although I can't tell you how to cope—or even how I cope—you might hear one sentence, one ritual, one strategy that on your darkest day can give you hope to keep going.

When I grieve for Violet, I am not only grieving the loss of her. I am grieving the loss of her future and all of the future memories we would never get to make. I am grieving everything that this experience has robbed me of. I grieve that for me, pregnancy will never be a blissfully happy and exciting time. I also grieve the person I was before I lost my daughter.

My experience with grief is related to the loss of my daughter, but I have friends who have experienced grief over long-term breakups and others over the loss of a parent who can relate and identify with some of my feelings. Experiencing life-changing grief is not something anyone wishes for but will most likely happen to each of us at some stage.

I have found grief to be an incredibly powerful teacher. It has completely rocked my perception of what should happen and has given me greater insight into the extreme struggles everyone faces when they deal with loss. However, there are odd upsides; not only has my grief journey provided incredible life lessons, but it has also given me a renewed appreciation for so much in life.

So, how do you walk forward with grief when it turns your world upside down?

For me, I began with a 'proactive' approach to tackling

my grief, which wouldn't surprise anyone who knows me. I was incredibly busy for the first six weeks after having Violet. Although I wasn't working at my job I certainly wasn't spending my days in bed or on the couch watching Netflix. Most days working on my healing and grief actually felt like a full-time job. I organised appointments for treatments that might make me feel good like facials and massages. I made time to catch up with people and scheduled meetings with others to discuss our journeys. Everything I was doing was incredibly beneficial, but it took me six weeks to realise it was too much too soon. What I most needed was time to feel everything I needed to feel. I needed time to be sad and sit in my feelings. I needed the time to just sit on the couch and watch Netflix.

Because I was so busy for the first six weeks, the adrenaline I had felt when I first left the hospital was still there. I hadn't paused to slow down. As the adrenaline wore off, the full onset of emotions began to unfurl. I was so unbelievably sad and feeling bad for feeling so sad. Everything began to feel harder.

I no longer wanted to catch up with people and discuss what I was going through. I didn't want to work on my writing.

After a week of feeling this way, I was pretty convinced I had postnatal depression. I didn't believe that I should be feeling so sad six weeks after saying goodbye. I thought I should have been feeling better. I didn't think receiving a text from a friend saying they were expecting their first baby should leave me crying every time I thought about it for the next two days. I didn't think seeing someone pregnant at the shops would all of a sudden make me want to leave.

I booked an appointment to see my GP for my six-week checkup and told her how I was feeling, and she asked me a range of questions. After thoughtful consideration, she told me that although everything I had experienced was incredibly traumatic, she just thought I was sad and grieving.

At my next psychologist appointment, I told her how incredibly sad I was and asked if I maybe did have postnatal depression. I was again asked various questions and was compassionately told that it was okay to feel so sad, I had just lost my baby. Although I know that postnatal depression is incredibly common after the loss of a baby, it was not what I was experiencing. I had merely underestimated the profound grief that I would feel.

There are so many sayings around grief. I remember even before saying goodbye to Violet finding information and articles on the stages of grief in the hope it would help me. I also loved reading the analogies about grief being like the ocean, or the weather or even a game of snakes and ladders. All of them relatively unpredictable and forever changing.

Looking back on the seven stages of grief that everyone talks about, I'm not so sure I went through them all and if I did, I don't know how long for. As time has continued, my feelings during my grieving process have been constantly evolving.

The other truth I have learnt about grief is that there is absolutely no timeframe. There is no guide that suggests how long each stage lasts or when you will begin to have some brighter days.

I was having dinner with a friend about four weeks after I said goodbye to Violet, and I told her I just wished that I knew when it would start to feel better. I just wanted a timeframe on when the heaviness in my chest would ease a little bit and when I would feel comfortable to re-enter the world. Her response resonated so deeply with me. She told me, 'If you had a date to work towards, you wouldn't feel everything you need to feel in order to heal. You would just focus on working towards the date.'

Five months after Violet's birth I had more sunny days and less rain. I learnt and accepted that it's as normal to feel sad in your grief as it is to have rainy days. Because grief can come in waves, I often found I could cope perfectly normally for hours or even days. I have continued to find it to be quite normal to have periods of calm and normality between waves of acute sadness.

The worst part about experiencing grief is that no one can say or do anything to take the pain away. It is yours alone to carry.

One of the most common things my friends and family would say to me was that they just wish that they could make it better for me. After my second session with my psychologist, she leaned forward and told me how badly she wished that there was something she could say or suggest that could ease some of my pain. Sadly, no one could change what happened and no one could bring back my baby.

I have worked harder at navigating and understanding my grief than at any other job I have ever had. If navigating grief were a professional sport, from the moment I left the hospital I immediately began training to play the game like a professional. I was pro-actively doing anything I could to help myself feel better. I sought help from medical professionals, I watched TED talks, I listened to podcasts and ordered books. Although a lot of what I was doing certainly did help, it also completely exhausted me.

Immediately after experiencing extreme loss, most people go through a stage of adrenaline where you deal with the immediate needs such as funeral arrangements, deciding what's happening with work and seeing everyone who wants to see how you are going. This sense of adrenaline takes a couple of weeks to leave and once it does the full extent of emotions take over. Usually this happens once people have stopped checking in as much and life starts to move on like normal.

Two months after Violet's death, I needed to learn to treat myself with compassion and kindness and acknowledge that like everyone else I was doing the best I could. Although this sounds incredibly simple, for me this really wasn't easy. For me to truly acknowledge that I was doing my best and let go of the crappy guilt that I felt every day of my grief, I had to find a strategy that worked.

My strategy was to treat myself like I would a good friend. Every time I felt guilt or criticised myself for feeling a certain way, I learnt to rephrase it as if for a friend.

Would I criticise or judge a friend for not wanting to see or hold a new baby after losing hers? Absolutely not. Would I question a good friend for having a sad day and wanting to lay in bed and watch Netflix all day? I would probably encourage it! Would I think less of a friend for not feeling able to return to work when they said they could? No, I would tell them to return when they are ready.

This small strategy was absolutely life changing for me and allowed me to take the time I needed to navigate through my grief journey.

As a couple, this was by far the most challenging and traumatic thing to ever happen to us. I remember one day only two weeks after losing Violet arguing with Chris about the fact he was going out. I could barely leave the couch and he was going to hang out with friends. I was so upset and angry.

From the start, we had been told by numerous hospital staff to be prepared that this would be a very challenging time for our relationship. We were told that surviving our loss might actually bring us closer together, but also had the possibility of a much harsher reality as we learnt to deal with our grief individually and as a couple.

Something I had to quickly realise was that we would often experience our grief at different times and express it in completely different ways.

That same day I was angry and upset with Chris for going out with friends, he was out for longer than he had planned as he had ended up enjoying himself. I became furious with him, we hadn't been apart in weeks and had spent most days together crying and looking at the photos of our girl. I couldn't understand how he could now manage to hold it together and be around other people.

I also knew that his friends wouldn't be talking about babies or children and after an initial bit of conversation Chris wouldn't be talking about Violet.

When he got home, I was inconsolable. I was so mad at him for leaving me and I was jealous he was able to enter back into the world so easily. Through my tears I had meanly told him I felt that he was moving on and no longer upset about Violet.

Chris is not the kind of person to get angry, he is always calm and kind, but he was furious with me. He couldn't believe I would think that let alone say it.

We realised we needed to sit down and have a conversation and communicate how we were both feeling. These conversations aren't new to us, they happen every few months in our relationship. There usually isn't an issue, we are both just open to discussing things we want to work on. The most recent discussion before all of this was when I discovered what the mental load was.

So, in our conversation we talked about how we were feeling and what we needed from one another. Chris explained that he needed the distraction of being around other people, he had cried all morning and just wanted to be distracted for a few hours. I didn't realise he had cried that morning and that made me feel better that he wasn't 'over it'. We agreed to be honest and open when we are down and to also talk about when we are feeling okay.

As I write this, I am six months into my new life with grief as a sidekick. So, what have I learnt that has helped me and could help you?

> I have learnt that days you think will be difficult are often okay and days that you expect to be relatively easy can have you hysterically crying.
>
> I have learnt that smiling and presenting myself positively in the world doesn't mean I am miraculously okay and 'over it' and that crying and having a bad day doesn't mean that I am not coping.
>
> I have learnt that you can function successfully in life and achieve career goals whilst also carrying heartbreaking grief.
>
> I have learnt that everyone grieves differently.
>
> I have learnt that my own grief has gifted me with the superpower to sit with others in their times of grief and sadness. Those who were able to sit with me were often the ones who had also had their own experiences of grief.
>
> I have learnt the importance of self-care and finding out what fills my cup and makes me feel good and ensuring I do as much of it as possible.

I have learnt that I can say no to anything that doesn't feel right or will require more energy than I can give.

To this day, I tell everyone that the best thing Chris ever did for me throughout all of this was cry in front of me and with me. Often, I will be in another part of our house, and he will come and find me for a hug and I know he has been crying. He also loves honouring and talking about Violet as much as I do and that has made my heart sing.

He has been my biggest support through this experience and my grief. We have attended parent support groups, remembrance ceremonies and awareness walks together. I have been unbelievably supported and encouraged in my various projects. I feel incredibly lucky to be able to say that becoming parents to our girl has brought us far closer than I could have ever imagined.

Losing Violet and experiencing life-shattering grief has been quite a journey. I continue to walk it daily, one step at a time. What I have learnt is not to run from my grief, but to make room for it and have the courage to accept it is now a part of me. I definitely believe that it is possible to find acceptance and strength on the other side of grief. I also know from experience that the way forward is by going through the grief, not around it.

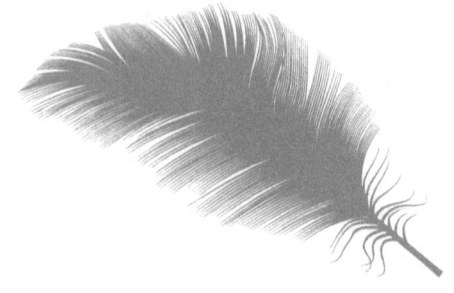

*I have learnt that you can function successfully in life and achieve career goals whilst also carrying heartbreaking grief.*

# CHAPTER SIX
# Say my baby's name

A few months after I had Violet I went out for coffee with a couple of friends. I hadn't seen them since well before I received the news that things weren't okay. I was sharing our story and about part way through, one of them put his hand on my arm and asked if we could have a break in the story because it was so intense. He asked if we could talk about something else as it was so heavy and reassured me that he was happy to come back to it but really needed the break.

We eventually came back to it, and I wrapped it up as quickly as possible and left out most of the details. I was a bit shocked that someone who I classified as a friend would react that way, but I was nowhere near as shocked as I was that night when I received a text message saying it was nice to catch up, but he was exhausted having to listen to what we had been through and had needed to lie down as soon as he got home.

The truth is, no one knows how to respond when someone in their life experiences extreme trauma or loss. No one wants to say or do the wrong thing and absolutely no one wants to further upset the person/people affected by the loss or trauma. Six months ago—pre-grief—I was exactly the same. I would awkwardly send a message and then probably never discuss it or bring it up again unless the other person started the conversation.

Losing Violet has completely changed that for me. My experience has forced me to evaluate and think about how I respond when others are going through a difficult time. It's probably good for all of us to pause and reflect, how do you respond when someone is going through something really challenging and difficult?

The coffee shop meeting with my friends wasn't the first time I'd been shocked by other people's reactions. There was the time a colleague told me that this happened to me because I am strong enough to deal with it. And the time a friend asked how long before I would get over it or when someone told me that their wife had miscarried but didn't make as big a deal out of it as I was.

I'm not recounting these moments to judge these people but because they do have a lasting impact on me. As much as I try to let the comments wash over my head, it's difficult when you're already trying to silence your own mental chatter—and then you're faced with other people's discomfort and insensitivities.

One of the most exhausting parts of my loss was dealing with other people's reactions to it. Especially in the first few months I spent so much time explaining myself and reassuring others. In my experience I came across three main categories of people: Those who celebrate your highs and are there for your lows too, those who love the drama of the situation, and those who care deeply and have no idea what to say, so they say nothing and 'give you space'.

The first category doesn't stop checking in after two weeks as they know that six weeks later you are still having a hard time (thank you!). The second category, generally, are people who before your loss you actually never had much to do with. They are completely distraught by your loss and will tell everyone they know, *Have you heard the terrible news?* They are also now sending you regular messages asking how you are and when they can drop off a lasagne.

The people that hurt me the most were those who completely ignored us and what we were going through. Those who continued to avoid saying Violet's name after I had asked them to.

What is the most difficult and traumatic thing you have experienced? What did you want from the people in your life? How would you feel if people just pretended it didn't happen?

I understand that it is uncomfortable, and everyone is terrified of saying the wrong thing so often they say nothing at all. My advice to anyone who finds themselves in that situation is to say something. Saying nothing makes it feel like you don't care, which is most often not the case.

I had a colleague approach me after my return to work and shared that although she felt she couldn't relate to much of my story as she isn't a mother herself, when I had asked everyone on my return to work to please not ignore me and what I have been through it instantly hit a nerve as when she had lost her mother two years prior the people who ignored her were the ones that hurt the most.

I had a good friend who I spoke to most days and even more

so when I was pregnant who didn't say a word when we lost Violet. The first conversation we had, she spent the entire time discussing the latest guys she was dating and didn't once ask me how I was. When she eventually came to our house, it was because she needed something. I know that all of this wasn't because she is cold and heartless, she is actually one of the kindest deepest souls. It was purely because she felt awkward and uncomfortable and had no idea what to say.

I have to remind anyone who feels that way, that the awkwardness you feel in the moment it takes to say something is nothing compared to the awkwardness and discomfort a bereaved person will carry for the rest of their lives.

But, for every uncomfortable comment, so much love has come our way too.

While there were a few reactions at times that had shocked and hurt me, overall, I was fortunate to have also been extremely supported by friends and family. Losing our baby opened us up to see a completely different side of people. We had been open and honest about everything we were going through in the hope it would make it easier for us and others, for some it helped and for others it had no impact at all.

Some of the nicest and most thoughtful messages and cards I received were the simplest. My nanna often just sent me texts of a heart emoji because she didn't know what to say to me but wanted me to know I was in her thoughts. The words *I can't begin to imagine what you are going through, but I am here for you* acknowledged us and the fact that unless you've experienced a similar loss you actually can't imagine it.

I had two kind friends message me and ask what I wanted, whether I wanted to be messaged every day or if I wanted my space. I loved that they asked me that as I didn't want any space, I really didn't want to be left alone. I had more than one person say that they hadn't contacted me because they were giving me space. I did need space but not weeks and weeks of it, if I couldn't respond to a message, I didn't.

In the days before my induction, one of the women I had reached out to on social media asked me if she could have my address as she wanted to drop off something before I went to the hospital. When we got home from the movies the next day, there was a large box full of various items on our doorstep. The goodies in the box were to help me and help create memories in hospital with our beautiful girl.

Some people's reactions were just confusing, especially from people I hadn't connected with in years. When I was still in the hospital, I had one lady who I hadn't seen or spoken to in five years message me with her exact availability that week to come over for coffee (she hasn't messaged again since).

I had people I went to high school with and don't think I had seen since contact me and ask if I wanted to catch up. I had an ex-colleague from over seven years ago who had recently had a baby tell me that because she was on maternity leave she had heaps of time to go for a walk with me. I honestly couldn't have thought of anything worse.

Most of these people I would probably have avoided if I saw them at the local shops and losing Violet didn't change that or make me suddenly want to be their best friend. I barely had the energy to see my actual friends, let alone all of the people who had randomly come out of the woodwork. I know that all of them had the best of intentions and were definitely just trying to be kind. But I didn't need their kindness at the expense of my wellbeing.

So, you can understand why I was a little nervous about what it would be like when I returned to work. The comments I might hear or whether people would take me seriously in my role or if my loss might change my relationships with colleagues.

After giving birth, one of the most common questions I was asked by people was *When are you going back to work?* I was asked it for the first time only five days after I returned from the hospital. That simple question that was probably just a casual conversation starter absolutely devastated me. I had given birth less than a week earlier and I was already being asked about my return-to-work plans (thankfully not by my actual workplace!). My body needed time to recover, let alone how I was feeling emotionally. To me this simple question was just another example of the lack of understanding people have around pregnancy loss. Absolutely no one would ask a mother with a living baby less than a week after she had given birth if she was going back to work.

Now, it was three months later, and the time had come to walk back into my workplace—back to the place I had hidden my pregnancy for five months, to the place where everyone knew the details of our story.

I had been back since my last official day of work four weeks after Violet's birth to share an update on our story, including small things they could do to support me, such as using her name and not ignoring what we had been through. But this was different—it was a milestone saying, *I'm ready to move forward with my life.*

Every mother feels trepidation going back after maternity leave, but my return came with so many layers of extra emotion. So many people asked me in those first few days if I was happy to be back and my honest response was, 'Not really.'

Being back at work felt like nothing had changed and everything was exactly the same, I found this so difficult as everything felt different to me. I felt like a completely different person. I also hated the feeling of moving on and leaving Violet behind. Going back to work felt like a really significant step and this was difficult for me to process and understand in the first few weeks.

The reactions I received when I returned to work were also incredibly mixed. Being back at work was the first time I had actually been surrounded by people who were not my close family and friends and I had to take a lot of what was said with a thick skin and big grain of salt.

On my first day back a lot of kind people said how nice it was to see me back. Many people looked the other way and completely ignored me. Some people who I had spoken to every day for over five years pretended I was transparent when I walked towards them. I was told by at least ten well-meaning people that it was probably good for me to be out of the house and doing something with my days. I have a feeling their image of me on maternity leave consisted of a pyjamaed woman rocking in a corner, crying all day and although sometimes that was how I spent my time, this book is evidence that I did other things too.

I had only one person say they were sorry for my loss and what I had been through. I know that they weren't comfortable in doing so, but it meant so much that they did. A handful of people shared their experiences and stories of loss with me. Included in those stories was some understanding and compassion, but there was also a very clear lack of understanding about what we had been through.

One man told me that his wife had had two miscarriages 'but didn't need to take off as much time as me'. Another told me that it would all be okay when I eventually had a real baby as I would 'be able to move on and forget all of this'.

Other people were just glad to have me back and doing my job. I had been there less than ten minutes before I was pulled aside and asked to help someone with an issue they had with another colleague. Another person also said that finding out I was pregnant and going through so much made a lot of sense in regard to some of the professional decisions I had made during that time.

It wasn't just the reactions of people I knew that were hard, but also the people I didn't know. Four weeks after Violet was born, I needed to attend a skin check follow-up appointment. I was really dreading going as the last time I was there I was pregnant and they had told me the hormones can often change your skin.

I was greeted by a heavily pregnant woman and taken into the consult room. As she turned towards the computer I tearily blurted out, 'I know it says I'm pregnant on there, but I just lost my baby.' As she was pregnant I expected a bit of sympathy, instead she said, 'Oh yeah, that happens, I'll let the doctor know.'

I was so shocked I said nothing after that. A few minutes later she went on to tell me she had had a miscarriage when she was twenty-four and people had told her that things happen for a reason and at least you're young. She told me how much she hated being told those things, but maybe I would like it. Suffice to say, I didn't.

I have learnt that what individual parents want and need to hear after they lose a baby is often different and unique to the couple. One couple at one of our pregnancy support group meetings mentioned the best card they received was a congratulations card as they felt that they deserved to be congratulated on the arrival of their baby. They said it was significantly more special than the condolence cards. To be honest, I couldn't think of anything worse.

When a couple of people commented 'Congratulations on your new bundle of joy' on our Facebook announcement post (I still don't think they had read it properly) I was horrified and deleted the comments immediately.

In saying that, there are some definite comments that we can all agree shouldn't be said to a person who has lost a baby. Many people who have experienced pregnancy loss have received some pretty horrific responses. I read some horrible stories in the Facebook support groups I'm in. One woman posted screenshots of a conversation between herself and a lady on Etsy. The lady on Etsy made Christmas decorations and the woman who had lost more than one baby had ordered some the year before for the babies she had lost. She contacted the woman as unfortunately she had lost two more babies during the year. The response was: 'LOL, another two? I can't keep up. Have you thought about getting a pet?'

The woman who kindly let me know this had happened to me because I was strong enough to handle it, reasoned that many others hadn't gone through it as they weren't as strong as me. I have mentioned this comment to lots of people, and others who have experienced other trauma such as cancer and other illnesses have told me they were told this by close family and friends.

I have also spoken to many people who have been told *Maybe you weren't meant to have children, Your baby is in a better place, At least you can fall pregnant, When do you think you will get over it? Have you considered adoption? When will you try again?* and my favourite of all *Everything happens for a reason*.

Even if you are a person who believes everything happens for a reason (like I am), telling a bereaved parent that is not a smart move. Because what reason could possibly exist for a baby dying?

In my experience, I have been fortunate enough that positive responses and support have far outweighed the negative. I have felt genuinely overwhelmed by the kindness of so many people in our lives. Losing Violet showed us both how unbelievably loved and cared about we are. I'll never forget the flowers that filled our house even before we had gone into hospital. The constant deliveries. How our fridge and freezer were bulging with delicious homemade meals. Or, how my mum and close girlfriend helped organise and pack my hospital bag with all the necessities as I didn't feel up to leaving the house.

We were given crystals and wellbeing packs full of our favourite foods, face masks and magazines. I received jewellery and candles and donations were made in memory of Violet. All of which was either sneakily dropped off on our doorstep or sent in the mail.

We had many people let us know that they supported our decision and that they would have made the same one in our position. I had a friend of a friend reach out who works in an organisation that supports children and adults with severe disabilities and extreme health concerns reassure me that what we did was the kindest and bravest thing we could do for our beautiful girl. She let me know she was happy for me to contact her if we ever questioned ourselves or our decision.

Most importantly, I'll never forget the messages and cards that included Violet's name. It made me feel she was acknowledged and loved.

Recently, I spoke to an old work colleague who confided in me that she had experienced a late-term miscarriage and after telling her how sorry I was for her pain and loss, I asked if her baby had a name. She burst into tears and told me that I was the first person to ask her that and make her feel that her baby and grief were acknowledged.

My favourite moments are when I get to share photos of Violet. Only two people asked me if they could see them, and it meant the world to me. For everyone else, I had to ask them first if it was okay to share her photos and await their response before showing them, like I was providing some sort of trigger warning. I understand why people don't ask and even my best friend said she really wanted to see pictures of her but didn't want to upset me by asking. Only one person said that they didn't want to see her pictures and when they eventually did see them at her celebration, they commented that she wasn't as scary looking as they thought she would be.

Although part of me can understand why it may be difficult for people to see photos of Violet, it doesn't make it any easier. How would you feel if someone told you they didn't want to see photos of your baby or children? Could you imagine questioning whether or not photos of your baby would be too confronting to have in your lounge room? Or imagine wishing you could share them on social media but knowing you can't without confronting or upsetting people.

So, how can you react in a healing way to support grieving parents?

Say their baby's name. There are actual books with that title written by bereaved parents, there are even poems written about it. Hearing Violet's name is magic to me, seeing it written in Christmas cards and text messages warms my heart.

Acknowledge what they have been through and continue to go through. Understand that their baby and loss is a part of their story and they will never move on or get over it.

Support grieving parents' decisions to not attend significant events. Be understanding if they find it difficult to be around your baby.

Think of them during significant events and milestones.

Two weeks after Violet's death I forced myself to go to the hairdresser's in the name of self-care. I had told them that I lost my baby via message when I booked, as they knew I was pregnant. When I anxiously arrived, I was greeted as per usual. Nothing was mentioned, and to be honest I was getting annoyed, because they knew what I had been through. Why weren't they saying anything?

At one stage I may have contemplated looking up other hairdressers as I wondered how they could be so insensitive. Then when I went up to pay at the end of my appointment, I was told it was a gift. They were so sorry for my loss and they hoped it helped make me feel better in some small way.

This is the thing about people's reactions—five insensitive comments can be washed away by an act of kindness from a stranger. A gift, a few words of acknowledgement. Hearing someone say your daughter's name.

Each of the people who showed us such incredible kindness gave us the greatest gift of all as they expected nothing in return. Although we know we cannot always return the kindness to those who bestowed it upon us during this time, we try our best to regularly pay it forward by sharing it with others in any way we possibly can.

*My advice to anyone who finds themselves in that situation is to say something. Saying nothing makes it feel like you don't care, which is most often not the case.*

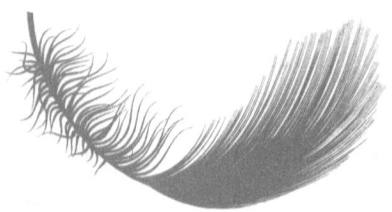

CHAPTER SEVEN
# A different kind of trauma

Six months after giving birth, I was beginning to realise that losing a very wanted and loved baby is so much more complex than I could have ever imagined. Prior to my experience I hadn't really understood the challenges I would continue to face after my immediate loss and experience. I knew I would be sad and I would grieve, but I didn't realise how many everyday tasks and moments would trigger me into sadness.

As the months went on, life became less scary and the triggers not only lessened but their impact wasn't as big and my recovery wasn't as long.

One morning, as I sat eating my breakfast, scrolling through Instagram and observing other people's lives from the outside, I realised that my grief was shifting every day—and my reaction to this traumatic experience was far from linear.

As time went on my attitude was slowly shifting—from being upset about the significant changes to my body to acknowledging how incredible my body has been for carrying and giving birth to my beautiful baby girl. I learnt how to manage different tasks that upset me, such as signing a birthday card, in a way that made me feel happy Violet was being acknowledged.

In all of the pamphlets and doctor's appointments I was told it would be normal to feel triggered into sadness and despair when you least expect it. That I may find reminders of my loss in the places I least expect them to be.

Some reactions I assumed were normal: seeing other pregnant women, other babies, experiencing various holidays and anniversaries, and going to the doctor's offices all may bring me to tears even when I feel strong. To me, all these were completely understandable and so much easier to cope with in some ways.

What I wasn't prepared for in addition to the above was how many random triggers I would experience after my loss. Things that seemed entirely harmless and wouldn't have required a second thought before Violet was born, now left me with watery eyes and shaky hands.

This included, but wasn't limited to: food, clothing, my body, signing birthday cards, having conversations with new people, family get-togethers, shopping centres, 'funny' mum memes, like, *I kept the children alive today*, going back to work, seeing old photos of myself, the smell of the body wash I used in hospital, babies who were due around the same time as Violet … and on the list could go.

One very significant shift was my relationship with, and attitude to, my body.

I had experienced all-day nausea for the entirety of my pregnancy. It began at six weeks and didn't disappear until I had actually given birth. I was also one of the unlucky ones who threw up most days, thankfully that finished at eighteen weeks.

I didn't actually realise during our time in hospital that my nausea had gone when I had given birth. I ate all of the hospital meals and enjoyed the delicious dairy snacks without a thought.

It wasn't until we came home and I had to think about what I wanted to eat that it really impacted me. I didn't develop an eating disorder, but I spent a few months with serious issues with food. My psychologist explained it to me as another element of guilt within my grief. I felt guilty that I was now able to eat everything and nothing made me sick. The options were endless surrounding what I could eat and it caused me serious anxiety. There was absolutely nothing I wanted to eat and, for a person who loves food, that is a big deal.

One lunchtime within the first two weeks of returning home from the hospital, Chris asked me what I wanted to eat, and I had a mini meltdown (not for the first time!). We'd had a lovely morning, so the outburst had come from nowhere and I hadn't seen it coming. But when he asked me the question 'What would you like to eat for lunch?' I felt anxiety rising in my stomach. *I don't know! Nothing! Everything!*

This simple question triggered me so much that I ended up lashing out at him. I can remember the look on his face as he struggled to digest the situation—and who can blame him? I was as confused by my reaction as he was.

I genuinely didn't know the pressure of that question was too much. Through endless discussion we learnt to rephrase the question and he would have to ask me if I would eat a certain food and I would respond with a yes/no answer.

When I went out for dinner with friends, I would not even

look at the menu, I just asked them to order the same for me.

Eventually, with the understanding and support of those around me, eating no longer provided a source of anxiety; as life began to return to a new normal so did my eating habits. I started taking on a more active role in cooking dinner by using a meal delivery service that delivered fresh ingredients and easy-to-follow recipes to our house. This gave me enjoyment in the food I was cooking and eating and was a really helpful and important part in moving forward.

Although in the first few months my close friends knew that I was struggling to decide what to eat, I hadn't really told anyone else. Then one day I saw a post another mum had written on social media stating how difficult she was finding the choice of eating food. She was reaching out and asking for suggestions on how to manage. I was a little bit further along in my journey and was able to share what had worked for me and to also acknowledge she wasn't alone. To my surprise lots of women had responded feeling exactly the same way.

I know that this reaction also isn't the same for everyone. In our support group another mum mentioned how as soon as she knew her baby wasn't okay, she had started drinking quite heavily and was actually seeking medical support to assist her with developing better strategies for coping with her loss.

Post-baby bodies are often a discussion topic, there are always magazine articles on celebrities bouncing back too fast or not fast enough. There are programs to help you get your pre-baby body back and friends make comments about how good one another look after having a baby. Unfortunately, none of this knowledge prepared me for the complexities of a post-baby body when you don't have your baby.

In the first few weeks my body was bouncing back way too fast and I was devastated that I barely looked like I had been pregnant. I now just looked like I overindulged on all the treats people had dropped off on our doorstep. I thought about all of those women desperate to bounce back after birth and all I wanted was to still be pregnant.

Although my body had begun to recover it was also completely unrecognisable to what it had been before. Even though Violet wasn't with me, my body reacted in the same way it would have if I had a living baby. My milk came in and it was another distressing reminder I was a mum without a baby in her arms.

None of my clothes fit and I had to keep wearing maternity clothes for far longer than I would have liked. Getting dressed each morning was another depressing reminder of my loss.

It took me four weeks to get up the courage to go to the shops to purchase some new clothes. I knew as soon as I entered the shopping centre I had made a mistake and should have taken someone with me for support. There were babies and pregnant people everywhere, they seemed to have multiplied since the last time I had been there.

I have to admit, shopping has never been an enjoyable experience for me. I get hot and bothered trying things on and just don't overly like anything about it. I much prefer to do my shopping from the comfort of my couch and online, but I was unsure about sizing and felt I should do it in person.

I was in the first shop for less than ten minutes. I had tried on two pairs of jeans, both a size bigger than I normally am and both were too tight. I was already hot and bothered and hating everything about it.

I went to one more store before deciding that I preferred to deal with wearing maternity clothes than the excruciating pain of trying to find clothes that fit and made me feel good.

It was only a couple of weeks after Violet was born when I realised I wanted—needed—to move my body more. But I knew I wasn't physically ready to sign up to a new gym membership and head back to a group class. I wasn't the same person I'd been back then. A happy compromise was walking my dogs each day, something I had to stop doing after giving birth and whilst my body recovered.

So, one morning, I set out—alone—on our regular walk around the block. Physically I felt so different, yet on my walk absolutely everything was the same. Nothing I could see had changed over the last few weeks.

I was halfway around the block on our walk and a woman stopped her car and asked if I could talk to her about the area. She was from America and looking at buying a house in our suburb. We spoke for a minute or two before she asked me how the schools were and if I had any kids. Without really thinking, I quickly said no kids. I felt so guilty once I realised my response. I felt like I hadn't acknowledged my baby girl.

I know since that conversation that it is okay to say I don't have children if I feel that the person doesn't actually deserve my full story. I have to judge the moment as it comes and I don't think it ever gets easier. I know people who have lost babies over twenty years ago who still feel guilty if they aren't acknowledged.

I continued walking my dogs each day as part of my routine and to ensure I was still getting out of the house. I slowly started trying to eat a bit better and not just for comfort. Once I returned to work, I also found myself a personal trainer and began to work out consistently.

Finding the right personal trainer was incredibly important for me. I had always done small group personal training classes and had actually developed a strong relationship with my personal trainer. I knew though that I didn't want to return to that, I was always relatively fit and could do all exercises given to us, I didn't want to go back to that group and have to explain the reason I could no longer do certain things.

It was for this same reason I didn't want to join a gym or bigger classes at the gym. I didn't want to disclose I had given birth three months earlier as I didn't want the awkward follow-up questions where I would inevitably make others uncomfortable when I told them my baby had died.

So, I decided to start with one-on-one personal training sessions. My goal and intention were to feel strong again and be consistent in whatever it was I chose to do, if I lost any weight, it would just be a bonus.

I went online and researched personal trainers in the area. I had narrowed my research down to three women and wrote them each an enquiry message. I briefly explained what I had been through and what my intentions were for working out.

I then made my decision based on what their responses to my enquiry message were.

One of the ladies unfortunately hadn't read my message properly as her response included the words 'Congratulations on your new bundle of joy'. When I clarified what I had written she was mortified but I was no longer interested in working out with her.

The response from the wonderful woman I had selected was: 'Hi Meagan, you've been through an incredibly tough time, and I think it's amazing that you are now feeling strong enough to start looking after yourself. I would love to help you feel strong again. When are you interested in meeting?'

I love my personal training sessions. On the wall there is a quote that says: 'It's not about perfect, it's about effort, and when you bring that effort every single day, that's where transformation happens. That's how change occurs.' I feel like that can be applied to all aspects of my life and healing journey.

Despite my progress, when it came to my body, it didn't mean I was immune to every other trigger. I froze with guilt one day when I had to write a congratulations card to a friend who'd recently had a baby.

I unexpectedly found myself sitting with a pen in my hand, panicking about how I was going to sign the card. I knew I needed to include our beautiful girl's name, but I didn't know how, so I just didn't include her. I felt incredible guilt about not including her as she was a part of our family, but I didn't feel I could write her name next to ours.

With a suggestion from my mum, I settled on including a little hand-drawn flower in the bottom right of the card. I spent almost an hour practising my flowers to work out how I wanted to draw it and it is something that I plan to continue to always do. Every time I write a card and put a little flower on it, it makes me feel proud that we are continuing to include Violet in our family story.

At Christmas time some people address their cards to 'Chris, Meagan and Violet' and those ones mean the most to me.

I love seeing her name in writing, so at Christmas on many cards I signed ours in the same way, including our girl.

After a friend's young child asked me if I had any kids and I responded with 'None at home', I felt awful not acknowledging Violet. I also silently hoped he wouldn't ask where they were if they weren't at home.

It's a lot easier to handle kids asking these questions as once you've answered, they have often moved on to the next point of interest. Most of the time, they also haven't paid that much attention to your answer.

Since losing Violet, meeting new adults for the first time causes me all sorts of anxiety as I know I will be asked what my job is, if I have a partner and if I have kids. Somehow in the first six months I managed relatively well to avoid that situation and aside from the random lady who asked me about our neighbourhood I hadn't actually been in an awkward situation where anyone had asked me.

I feel much less nervous about answering that question as time has moved on and know that my answer will depend on what sort of conversation I am willing to have at the time.

I also found watching television or a movie a total minefield. You never know when a character is going to be pregnant or if there is going to be a plot relating to babies. I did find watching trashy television a good distraction but, even if the TV show you are watching is pretty much guaranteed child free, the ads aren't.

One day I was watching *The Bachelorette* knowing that the most extreme reference to children would be people saying they want them or already have them. During the first ad break there was an ad for nappies that turned me into a total blubbering mess. I watched the little baby on the screen crying and moving their arms and legs around and it made me so unbelievably sad that I had never got to see Violet move or hear her cry.

But I did feel my traumatic reactions lessening, or at least shortening—which was a relief. I discovered that I was able to regroup pretty quickly when the show was back on and I was watching the men battle over who got a private chat at a cocktail party.

Then the next lot of ads came on and there was a preview for the new season of *One Born Every Minute*.

In the preview, an exhausted mother had her beautiful baby placed on her chest with a congratulations from the midwife, her partner was leaning on the bed next to her with so much love and admiration. They both had tears in their eyes and were clearly overwhelmed with love.

Watching that fifteen-second commercial, my heart broke as my experience of meeting Violet couldn't have been more different. Our tears were because our baby wasn't alive and there weren't any words of congratulation to be heard.

In some of the online support groups there are regular posts made with trigger warnings to other loss mums. They will mention the show and what occurs in the episode as a warning.

One thing I have noticed in my viewing is that I am not interested in anything that doesn't leave me feeling good or some sort of joy. I have probably always preferred movies and shows like that, but it is now almost required.

For me, life can feel heavy, so I don't want to watch a TV show or movie that is going to leave me feeling the same way.

For some reason that same rule doesn't apply to the books I read and if it is a page turner, I am here for it.

Children with the same name as my baby was something I hadn't given any thought to as being a trigger. It occurred to me for the first time when I was standing in the baking section of the supermarket, trying to work out what icing I needed to buy to make the cookies for Violet's memorial. A little girl ran up to where I was standing and her mum called out to her from further down the aisle, 'Violet, make sure you don't go too far.' I was completely caught off guard. I couldn't stop staring at the little blonde-haired girl, wondering what she was like and if my Violet would have been like her. I managed to pull myself together by the time the mum caught up and smiled politely so I didn't look too strange.

It happened again at the Sands organisation fundraiser walk where we remembered our babies who have been lost. At the end the of the walk, the lady running the event asked her daughter, Violet, to come to the stage and help pull out the tickets. Once again, I was caught off guard and my heart started beating a little faster and then, like most unexpected triggers, it passed.

There are also triggers that don't cause an immediate reaction or response.

Someone I knew who was due to have a baby two weeks before me posted the arrival of their beautiful baby girl on Facebook. I looked at the post and immediately looked away. I didn't cry but I didn't write congratulations or anything else.

The next morning, I woke up with a black cloud hanging over me, everything felt heavy, unfair and sad. It took me half a day to realise that I was deeply upset she had given birth to a beautiful and healthy baby girl and instead of getting ready to welcome my own baby girl I was wearing her ashes within the ring on my finger.

All of these triggers, whether they get an immediate response or cause more long-term sadness, are hard to deal with and often completely unexpected. They are all just another challenging and difficult reminder of losing a baby.

There are also things that prior to my experience I would have never considered or understood. Someone I know who experienced the loss of their baby twenty-three years ago told me that the triggers and reminders don't get any easier, you just get better at dealing with them.

She told me that when her friend's children turned eighteen and got their licences it was another small reminder that her baby never got that opportunity. It didn't have her in instant tears or in a deep sadness, but it was a reminder of her loss.

One of the most important parts of my journey has been knowing that I am not alone. Knowing I am not alone in my grief but that there are also other people who find it weird hearing their baby's name said aloud or knowing that they have also found eating food difficult.

When I began Violet's Gift it was purely a fundraising campaign, but it didn't take long for it to evolve into something even greater. I had so many people reach out and thank me for helping make them feel less alone.

I eventually began sharing the stories of others regularly on our social media pages. People would send me what they had been through, and I would edit it and post it online as a quote.

Although each story was unique in its own way, there were so many elements that we could each relate to. Almost all of the people who had shared their story, including Chris, had mentioned how isolating and lonely their experience was. Each of the people who had shared said how quiet and how traumatic it had been and continued to be.

In sharing their stories and writing this book, I hope that it helps others feel less alone but also helps those who have never experienced the loss of a baby understand the complexities and different types of ongoing trauma that exist.

I look back on myself six months ago and how far I have come, and I am so incredibly proud. I want to tell myself and anyone that is there that it is crap, but you will be okay. The triggers will lessen, you will emerge stronger than you ever could have imagined possible.

About six weeks after I started sessions with my personal trainer, I woke up one morning really not wanting to go—everyone has days where their fitness motivation is lacking. But I forced myself into my gym gear and made my way to our session anyway, knowing I'd feel disappointed later if I hadn't. After a tough workout with my trainer, we were sitting on mats stretching when she turned to me and said, with admiration not sympathy, 'I bet Violet is watching you now thinking "look how amazing and strong my brave mum is".'

For me, this was a milestone moment I'll never forget.

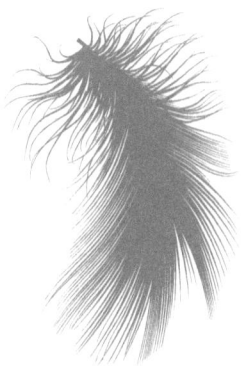

*The triggers will lessen, you will emerge stronger than you ever could have imagined possible.*

## CHAPTER EIGHT
# Redefining me

Who am I?

This is the question that sprung into my mind as I sat at our dining table the week that Chris returned to work. It had been three weeks since he took paternity leave—three weeks that we'd spent organising, crying, talking and sitting in silence when we needed to. After three weeks, I was completely exhausted and surprisingly grateful to have some time alone.

I hadn't given myself any time to process what I had gone through physically, emotionally and spiritually. I needed to slow down and take time for myself. I needed to work out who I wanted to be and what I wanted to do with my life.

That is how I ended up in a psychologist's office.

Getting to know myself and focusing on who I wanted to be is not something that began when I fell pregnant. It is something I spent the majority of my twenties working on. I have read countless self-help books, attended many different talks, listened to so many self-development podcasts, attended various weekend courses and made deep connections with others. I have been doing the work on who I am for years.

But for the first time in my life, I really needed to draw on everything I had ever read, learnt and heard and put it into action not only to better myself as a person but in order to survive the trauma of the situation I found myself in.

I always feel better when I focus on self-work and I have always found the more time I spend on it the more it allows me to show up more fully in all aspects of my life. In saying that, there have also been many times in my life where I have found myself too 'busy' to do the self-work. I have had too much on my schedule to fit in the meditation or reading and I have suffered for it. I am a better person when I look after myself first, we all are.

Well, now I was on maternity leave I couldn't use the 'no time' excuse anymore.

Before I was pregnant, seeing a psychologist had been incredibly beneficial to me at different stages of my life. I didn't consider going back to one of my previous psychologists as I wanted an expert in baby loss. I also wanted to work with someone who didn't already know me.

I decided to book an appointment with a lady recommended to me by my GP who specialises in pregnancy and infant loss. I googled her and read all of her credentials and all of the impressive boards she was on and the groundbreaking research she had been a part of. For the first time in weeks, I felt excited to book an appointment with someone so impressive.

And, I had a LOT to talk about and try to unravel.

Wife. Daughter. Sister. Friend. Educator. Leader. These are the labels that have been placed on me, both by myself and by society. For a period of time, I also had the label of expectant mother and was so looking forward to having the label of mother (which I know I still have). I now also have the not-as-flattering new label of bereaved mother.

When there are changes to the way you define yourself or imagine defining yourself it is incredibly confronting and anxiety inducing.

Our pregnancy journey and entry into parenthood had rocked me completely. I was no longer the person I thought I was going to be. I didn't like the label of bereaved mum and didn't want to be defined by it. I am Still A Mum.

But in all honesty, I no longer desired to be defined by any of those labels. I needed more. I needed to work out who I was without the labels. I didn't even think about inviting Chris to the appointment, and he didn't ask to be included. I think we both knew; this was a step I needed to take—alone!

My heart raced as I got in the elevator and selected the floor the psychologist was located. I checked my confirmation email about ten times, making sure I was at the right place. I was nervous but also excited to tell my story. I was also trying not to have preconceived expectations about this being a 'magic fix'—but I secretly hoped it might be!

At my first appointment, Emma opened the door with a smile and invited me into her nicely styled office. Luckily for me, I clicked with her instantly. As we sat facing each other with a box of tissues between us, I cried solidly for the whole hour as I told her from start to finish what we had been through.

At the end of my retelling, I waited for her to speak and the first thing she did was acknowledge our unbelievably traumatic story and how sorry she was that this was our reality. This was the first time the full magnitude of everything we had been through was reflected back to me.

My story was sad.

And I was sad it had happened.

At the end of the session, she asked what I wanted to gain from seeing her. I instantly replied with strategies to help make me feel better. Unfortunately for me, she said that there were no strategies that could make me feel better instantly. My homework: Make time every day to sit in a newly created space in my home—to just be.

I was also given permission to wallow in my grief. During certain times, I listened to incredibly sad and heartbreaking songs and bawled my eyes out. I also wrote in my journal to Violet and filled in pages in her memory book.

Journaling is something I have never been very good at. I have always had positive intentions when I start off writing in a nice new journal, but I often feel awkward and forget to write in it. I explained this to a friend who mentioned it as something to try and she suggested I use it as a way to communicate with Violet and just write to her. For me, that changed everything and I obsessively wrote in it every day—sometimes more than once!

When I wrote to Violet each time, I made sure to note down what I was grateful for that day. These were not big things like health or family, these were small things like a thoughtful text, seeing a butterfly or having a yummy treat.

'It can help to find reasons to be grateful every day,' my

psychologist said.

Well, when your child has died this can be easier said than done—but I persisted!

I found that focusing on the little things each day was crucial for me to be able to bring some joy back into my life. If I paused to look at the big picture and focus on the big things I had coming up or could look forward to, there really wasn't a lot. In recording the small things to be grateful for, I found myself looking for them each and every day. I would go for a walk and stop to look at the beautiful flowers and enjoy the feeling of the breeze on the back of my neck. I found myself, for the first time in my life, literally stopping to smell the roses.

I also rediscovered the magic of random acts of kindness and how doing something for someone else can make us feel really good. I began by writing a list of people I was grateful for during our experience and thought about what I could do for them. I had some beautiful cards made with Violet's hand holding my finger and I sent some to the midwives at the hospital and the sonographer. I also sent a card and a spa voucher to our doctor.

Let's be honest … when your world is ripped apart you will try *anything* to make yourself feel better. It's very easy to think mindfulness and even counselling is too hippy and a waste of money, until you've hit rock bottom and realise you just can't pull yourself up on your own.

In the first months after Violet's death, I'd have remortgaged our house to pay a magician for a bag of magic beans if I thought it would take my pain away—or bring her back!

This is also why, three weeks after Violet's death, I booked a reiki session. It wasn't my first taste of energy healing. Three years earlier, I had completed a two-day course to learn about alternative healing methods to cope with anxiety. Back then, reiki wasn't so mainstream and was definitely seen as a little bit woo-woo by my friends. But as I said, desperate times call for imaginative measures. And, after losing Violet, I was open to looking into anything for relief—and answers.

I honestly have no idea if the reiki session actually helped. But it did give me an opportunity to slow down, be in the moment and stop thinking for a little while.

I also started dabbling in tarot cards (which didn't tell me anything I didn't already know …). And I thought over and over about a conversation I had with my nanna about a dream she'd had just before I was pregnant: She woke up startled to see my grandad who was no longer with us standing at the end of the bed. On the table next to him was a pair of pink booties, an envelope and the time on the clock said 1.40 am. Six months later, Violet—our little girl—was born at exactly 1.40 am.

After Violet was born, I really got into looking for signs. I read two books about them and had regularly started seeing what I hoped were signs from my baby telling me she was okay. When the candle flame would flicker or I would come across a feather, I would tell myself it meant she was close by.

A few weeks after coming home from the hospital, I planted a whole heap of violet flowers in two big pots in our front yard. The next day when I left the house to go for a walk there was a butterfly on the flowers. I took a photo and remembered to write it down in my journal.

The next day I went for a walk and looked for the butterfly and was sad to see it wasn't there, but on my return it was back.

The same thing happened for a third day, and I completely lost it. I couldn't stop crying looking at the same butterfly sitting on my baby's flowers.

Chris began seeing 11:11 constantly and asked me to look up the meaning. When I did one of the meanings said *A deceased loved one is sending you a message.* We would both often see it and once I shared it with my mum, she saw it too.

I know that many people will think that seeing and believing in signs like this is silly and strange, most of these things could be explained as a coincidence. But I have learnt to believe as it has given me incredible strength and comfort to think my baby is always with me.

Those hours with my psychologist became special, sacred times. Sometimes, it felt to me like everyone's lives were moving forward, including my own. But, for that one hour I was allowed to cry and share my darkest thoughts. I was given permission to break down and not have to hold it together anymore. She was the one I confided in about the ups and downs I felt; how hurt I was by people's insensitive comments and my mixed feelings about returning to work after maternity leave.

It's an odd relationship you have with any therapist, because you know it won't last forever—you don't want it to either! You want to know that one day, you'll be 'fixed' enough to go it alone, but you also don't want to give up that person who can reassure you, comfort you and stop you feeling quite so crazy.

And then it happened …

Seven months after our first meeting, she suggested that I didn't really need her anymore, unless of course I wanted to continue. She was breaking up with me. I had found a new version of myself by visiting her. Stronger but also softer, more hopeful but also more in touch with my heartbreak, rawer but more resilient than ever.

Getting to know myself again hadn't uncovered a simple answer—but it had made me more accepting of all the sides of me!

2 August 2019
Hi Baby Girl,

Today it has been two weeks since you were born and we got to meet you.
Fridays are bittersweet as it was the day you were one week older. Fridays are the day I would send weekly updates on what size fruit/vegetable you were.

Today we should be celebrating being twenty-five weeks pregnant.

I don't want to always focus on the shoulds and should bes. So I will try to reframe today and say we were lucky enough to meet you and hold you two weeks ago.

It feels so long ago, but also like no time has passed at all.

I am currently lying in bed with Charlie and Tilly and we heard a bird hit the window. We looked it up and it said—it's an omen that could mean:

Someone in heaven is sending you a message.
Change is coming soon.

It also said something about money, but I ignored that bit.

Anyway, beautiful girl, I am having lunch with your Nanny and Great Nan today and I am sure we will talk all about YOU.

I love you so much Violet Grace.
Love, Mum xxx

# CHAPTER NINE
# A Grandparent's grief

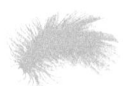

It's funny, I can't even remember messaging my mum on the morning I took the tablet that would end my pregnancy. But she will never forget it, or so she told me when I interviewed her for this book shortly after what would have been Violet's due date.

'You called me, the morning you took the tablet,' she recalled. 'It could have been a text. I just remember your words, "I can't do it". That was heartbreaking. Not just for me, for all of us, for you. Because I put myself in your shoes and I can't imagine being in that situation and having to do it either.'

Both sets of our parents were so excited to become grandparents. They were excited to have someone special to spoil with love and affection.

It's many mothers' hope for their children that they will be able to experience becoming a parent themselves. Watching your daughter-in-law or daughter's belly grow, their excitement and their joy. Having grandchildren is supposed to be one of the most cherished joys of growing older. So, how does it feel when the fairytale doesn't go to plan?

In the past twelve months, my relationship with my mum has shifted, been tested, grown and strengthened in so many ways. Grief does that to any close relationship!

In addition to Chris, my mum has been my biggest support person. I spoke to her on the phone or saw her almost every day during my pregnancy and in the initial months that followed.

My mum has ridden the highs and lows of each and every stage of my pregnancy. Each time we received a positive test result or news we didn't want to hear she was there. She remained hopeful with us up until that final phone call. She was also the first person, aside from the medical team, Chris and me, to meet Violet, her granddaughter.

'When we first walked into the hospital and I could see this tiny little bundle, just a tiny little bundle … I don't think I realised how tiny she would be either,' she remembered. 'She was perfect, but tiny. Meeting Violet and going through all those other things with you was hard, but that one phone call, hearing you say, "I can't do it," was the hardest.'

After giving birth and saying goodbye to Violet, I would call Mum each day and relive each and every moment of what I had been through and how I was feeling. At times I would speak to Mum about my feelings more than to Chris because I was more worried about upsetting him.

But this isn't only our grief. Many pregnancy loss resources say that grandparents experience a double grief. The grief of losing their grandchild and also the grief of who their son or daughter was before this occurred.

This is why it was so important for me to include a chapter here dedicated to grandparents—to my own parents' coping mechanisms and how they've tried to process our new reality as they have supported me through my own heartbreak.

It wasn't an easy conversation to have with my mum.

As she said, 'There were things we didn't see, conversations I didn't hear, a side of the story I was too buried in my own grief to observe. As your mum, I couldn't fix any of it, which is what a mum tries to do. We didn't know what to expect of Violet, I didn't know what frame of mind you would be in or Chris. It was just the unknown. It's all unknown to us, it's not something you go through. We don't want to go through it ever again, but I think as grandparents and your parents, we were just, I just wanted to get there, to the hospital. I just wanted to get there to make sure you were okay.'

When you're immersed in your own grief, you can become quite selfish—I can say that because I've been there! I've spoken to so many women and men who've experienced some kind of loss and many of them can look back and see how they became closed off and self-absorbed in a way. We are so busy thinking about our own emotional survival that considering other people in our lives—especially our close friends and family—can take up too much energy.

In the early days after Violet's death, I didn't think about the emotional burden my mum was carrying, or how my constant phone calls might have drained her. I needed her. I knew she wanted to help me in any way she could.

Our relationship was one-sided though. I had nothing to give her and I needed all the support I could get. We were both coming to terms with the 'new normal' of our lives.

'I just wanted your pregnancy to be a good pregnancy,' she

said. 'I didn't want you to be sick and I didn't want you to be … I wanted everything to go right.'

Similarly, to Chris and me, when we first discovered we were pregnant, she assumed that we'd all be welcoming a baby before Christmas—a healthy, happy, additional member to our family.

It breaks my heart to think of the milestones my mum endured instead. Waiting for her daughter to give birth to a baby that wouldn't be breathing, meeting her lifeless granddaughter for the first time and coping with the question marks over what would come next for me.

It would be easier in a way to never have considered the impact on my parents. It certainly would have been easier not to have asked them about it. But, when my editor, Amy, suggested that I interview my mum about her journey—and her grief—I knew that I had to do it, no matter how hard it would be.

We decided to go out for lunch and make a day of it—mum and I. First we went for a beach walk and then to my favourite café.

This café was my go-to when I was on maternity leave. Once a week I would go for a beach walk and then have breakfast at the café and write in my journal to Violet. On my first visit they served my muesli with decorative violets, and I knew it was a sign.

We enjoyed our walk and our breakfast together, both a bit nervous for what was to come next. We had agreed that we would go back to my house for the interview as neither of us knew how we would feel or react.

When it came to unearthing her memories, my labour—and what came after—seemed like a good place to start.

Amazingly, when I remember my mum meeting Violet, she was smiling.

'Yes, because Violet was peaceful,' she remembered. 'And I didn't know, I suppose we didn't know what condition she was going to be in. And so that would also affect you, I'm guessing, but as it was, she just looked beautiful. And peaceful like she was sleeping.'

I thought she'd only have negative memories of that moment, but quite the opposite was the case.

'For me the thing that stood out was how much love you could have for a little girl that's not even here,' she said. 'I walked out of that hospital, and I didn't want to leave her. I just felt so much love for Violet. And I didn't expect to feel that connection, when we can't actually make a connection as we grow.'

Unlike my grief, which felt like it hit instantly—and even began before I gave birth—my mum confessed that her grief was frozen, postponed, put on pause. I was the priority.

'I think I'll grieve for Violet later,' she said. 'My first concern was for you.'

It was hard to hear how my mum's own grief emerged, in unexpected moments just like mine did. How she had broken down in tears, just the night before, when Chris and I had gone to the shops to buy Violet a gift to donate to a local charity for Christmas, and she realised she hadn't got her anything.

How she felt she still couldn't shake the sadness she carried, even though so many people said it would lessen over time.

'The worst thing that could ever happen to anyone has happened to you,' she told me. 'The loss of a child would be my worst thing and that's happened. And then you, as your mum, I wanted to help you get through that.'

Until I sat down and asked Mum some of these questions, I didn't realise how helpful it was for her that I was talking to her constantly. I felt it must have been a bit of a burden, but I was thankful for her support. I was surprised when I interviewed her, and she confessed she loved my phone calls.

'Because talking to you is actually helping me as well,' she said. 'I think telling me everything helps me. Because if you kept it to yourself then I'd be sitting there thinking, *Oh no, what's she going through.* You just put it out there. So, then I knew how you were at any given moment, because we talked all the time.'

What an amazing gift Mum had given me. In that moment, I was so happy I'd interviewed her. Although I still felt guilty for leaning on her so much, on some level, I could understand how our constant conversations were better than an awkward silence. And I knew that I could continue to call her if I needed to—even if I needed to less as time went on.

We talked about a LOT during that interview: how grief could have pushed us apart, what I hoped for in the future, the pressure grief sometimes put on my relationship with her, and a lot of thoughts I couldn't share with anyone else—because I knew she'd never judge me.

I hope that my mum found our interview as therapeutic as I

did, even though it was hard to raise these topics. As I stopped recording the conversation on my phone, I felt happy. The conversation was emotional but it was also nice for me to hear how much Violet is loved by people other than Chris and me.

My relationship with my mum has changed and strengthened, as time moves on we are enjoying life together again. It is nice having conversations not solely around how I am feeling and about Violet, although I must admit she is mentioned or discussed still in some way. But we no longer relive the same story over and over again with every conversation we have. We are able to celebrate other aspects of our lives and make fun memories. Birthdays and other milestones aren't what we had anticipated, but we both work hard to ensure they are a new or different kind of special.

I know that if I am ever fortunate enough to be pregnant again or have any more children, Mum will be an incredibly important part in that. She will also continue to play an important part in helping keep Violet's memory alive and acknowledged.

I also realise that we are the lucky ones whose bond has been strengthened by grief. I know that losing a baby can actually fracture families.

In my support group, one of the women shared how excited her mum was for her first grandchild when she shared the news early on in her pregnancy. Her mum called regularly and began purchasing small items for her grandchild. At her twenty-week scan the woman received news and results that no one wants to hear, her baby was incredibly unwell. After she shared the heartbreaking news with her mum, she no longer heard from her.

Her mum answered her calls when she shared an update after an appointment, but she no longer called or talked about her grandchild.

This continued through to when she had to give birth at twenty-five weeks and her mum told her that coming to the hospital was too emotional for her.

This woman shared with the group that she was worried her relationship would never be the same again, her mum wasn't there for her when she needed her most. She also expressed that if she is fortunate enough to have other children, she doesn't want her mum to excitedly be there for every step of that journey when she wasn't there for the birth of her son.

So, what is my advice for grandparents whose granddaughter or grandson is born perfect but lifeless? I can only speak from my own experience, but I'm happy to share my insight if it helps a family to find solace.

As a grandparent you may feel many of the strong and unexpected emotions bereaved parents might feel but may question whether your feelings are as justified. You might also feel that it takes longer to grieve, like in my mum's case, because you are putting so much energy into helping your child first.

The most important thing my mum did to help me throughout my entire journey with Violet was to be there. She answered every phone call, messaged regularly and came over when I needed her. All I wanted to do was talk about Violet and she was there to listen. Mum also regularly offered to help in any way she could, which included making meals and preparing my hospital bag.

It is so important as a grandparent, close friend or relative to also continue to make contact. It made such a difference to me to know that we weren't alone and that others were thinking of Violet and were also there for us months after she was born.

Using your grandchild's name and ensuring they are included in your family is so important. Mum has photos of Violet printed on the wall and Nanna has a little angel figurine in amongst all of the photos of her great grandchildren, as well as a photo of our family displayed with all of the other family photos. These acknowledgements help bereaved parents know that others love and care about their baby like they would if they were alive.

It's also important that they are included when you say how many grandchildren you have. If Mum continued to have more grandchildren and she didn't include Violet when people asked how many she had my heart would absolutely break. It would feel like she didn't feel her life mattered.

Remembering special days, birthdays and anniversaries is also incredibly important. Prior to Violet's due date and as Christmas approached, Mum asked me what I wanted to do and needed. Originally, she wasn't going to message me on Violet's due date as she didn't want to interrupt our weekend away, but I told her that in my mind I would probably think she didn't care or had forgotten, which was obviously not the case. I'm incredibly glad we were able to have that conversation.

On Christmas Day my mum also put a small packet

of chocolate biscuits that were a pregnancy craving in my Christmas stocking and I think it was probably one of my favourite gifts as it acknowledged my baby.

As a grandparent, you might find that you also have to be aware that your child may be sensitive to other people's words and actions. You may say something that is misinterpreted or upsets your child. I am thankful that this didn't happen often and when it did, my mum allowed me to feel what I needed to feel and didn't get defensive or create any sort of issue out of it.

I think in all of this advice, the best thing to do if you're really not sure is to ask. Ask your child what they need from you, ask if they want you to use their baby's name, ask if they want to celebrate them on milestone days. Don't assume anything, because you might avoid saying their baby's name in hope of not upsetting them, but in fact you not saying it actually makes them think you don't care.

In the words of Mum, 'We are grandparents, and I would never say we weren't. My granddaughter was born beautiful yet still.'

*We are so busy thinking about our own emotional survival that considering other people in our lives—especially our close friends and family—can take up too much energy.*

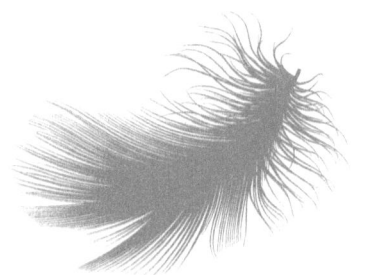

# CHAPTER TEN
# Life in limbo

'Surprise, we're having a baby!'

As my close friend and her husband broke their happy news, the crowd of people—friends and family members, gathered in their living room—all immediately broke into applause and congratulations. I feigned surprise too. Although, of course, I'd known already.

My friend, Sarah, had called me a couple of weeks earlier to tell me that she and her husband were planning to share that they were expecting their first baby at her birthday party that I had been invited to—and to give me a get-out clause.

'You don't have to come,' she'd said. 'I totally understand how difficult it might be for you.'

The truth is, since knowing about their surprise announcement I wasn't planning to go. I was apprehensive about attending the party for many different reasons, I was worried about how everyone's excited reactions would make me feel. I was also worried about how people would react to me being there, would those who knew about my experience watch me to see how I responded? Would I be able to respond appropriately, or would I get unexpectedly emotional? These were the sorts of questions on my mind.

When I heard about the party, I told my friend that there was a high chance that I may not go and that it would need to be a last-minute decision based on how I was feeling on the day. This was a wonderful coping mechanism I have used with most social events since losing Violet. It has given me an out and relieved so much pressure from me around feeling like I have to attend something because it's the right thing to do.

But here I was. And amazingly, I was even happy for them (mostly!). I arrived at the party with another close friend, Bec, who also knew about the surprise. I was incredibly nervous walking in the door of the party and just hoped that they would get the announcement over with quickly before I changed my mind about being there.

The day the party arrived I felt okay. I genuinely felt that I could go and be there for the excitement of the pregnancy announcement. I had one close friend with me as a support and I was okay.

Once they began the speeches and thanked everyone for coming, I braced myself for the announcement and reaction, but it really didn't upset me like it might have even a month earlier. After the emotions of the announcement, I hugged and congratulated the couple and joined in their happiness.

Bec and I even discussed how amazing it was that I was able to attend a surprise pregnancy announcement party at all. Even though my heart still ached to think of this new life growing in my friend's belly, I had to acknowledge how far I'd come. Despite my mixed feelings, I did feel incredibly proud of myself.

It certainly didn't have zero impact on my emotions, but I

found after five months it hurt less and I was able to rebound quicker. I am not sure I could have done it any earlier and it definitely wasn't always this way.

For roughly four months, I felt like I'd been living in limbo. This is what I had realised one day as yet another friend announced the news of her pregnancy to me.

Since Violet's birth, I had felt like I was standing on the outside watching everyone enjoy their lives while mine felt like it had completely fallen apart. All around me, people were having parties, getting married, having kids, falling pregnant and living their best lives. For me, everything hurt. I felt like I would never be one of those happy people who could join in on celebrations again.

For a while there, it was all too much. How could people be so full of joy and happiness when I was so miserable? I didn't begrudge anyone their happiness, but I certainly couldn't be a part of it.

Looking back on that time, I can see that grief had disconnected me, frozen me, put me in a box with a lock, no key. I didn't feel like I could join in on life. I didn't want to celebrate in other people's lives.

But, like every lesson I'd learnt from grief, that slowly began to change.

Sometime between Violet's due date on 15 November and just before Christmas, I had begun to feel like I was able to—gently—join in again. I felt happier and lighter. I still continued to carry my grief, but it had started to shift slightly and no longer felt all consuming. I began to feel less guilt for enjoying myself like I had in the initial months after Violet died. Socialising and celebrating important milestones didn't terrify me quite as much as they once did.

What I struggled with most during my pregnancy was not the uncertainty of our situation but hiding what was going on and pretending I was living my life as normal. All of our close family and friends knew what we were going through, and we stuck with our decision not to share it with others until we had a clear idea of what was happening. I don't regret our decision as we really didn't need the advice or input of well-meaning colleagues or distant friends.

There were also so many pregnancy announcements during this time and the mothers were all due two or three months after me. I plastered a smile on my face and congratulated each person on their exciting news and asked questions about how they were feeling, their due date, or if they were finding out the gender. On the inside my heart hurt, I just wanted to be able to share in the excitement, I wanted everyone to know I was expecting my first baby too.

I remember one day standing in the lunchroom, trying to hide my stomach behind a friend whilst we listened to another pregnancy announcement. Once it was complete, a lady I didn't know that well came up to me and said, 'I thought that was going to be about you.' I brushed it off and pretended I had to get to a meeting. I was assured by my friend that I hadn't given anything away, but I still felt sick.

When I was nineteen weeks pregnant one of my close

friends had her hen party and at the last minute I had made the decision not to go. I didn't know how to be in a room full of excited women who were living their best lives. There were going to be three other pregnant women there and I didn't know what to say to anyone. Was I supposed to tell them I was pregnant but didn't know if my baby was okay?

How would you react at a hen party if one of the other guests said that to you? You can pretty much guarantee that would bring the mood down.

At this stage I also couldn't get away with hiding my stomach at the party; unless I wore a coat and scarf for the duration of it people would have known I was pregnant.

Four weeks after Violet was born it was that same friend's beautiful destination wedding. I had my flights and accommodation booked but decided just before that I couldn't go.

This was the most exciting moment of their lives, it was my worst. The thought of being surrounded by happy families, pregnant women, babies and children in a beautiful destination felt like it would have been torture for me. I didn't have enough strength to fake it and pretend I was okay for the sake of everyone else.

Instead, I sat on the couch bawling my eyes out, looking at the beautiful photos everyone was posting on social media. As much as I wished I could have been there to celebrate with my friends, I know that I had made the right decision.

About five weeks after we said goodbye to Violet, I received a kind and well-thought-out text message from a colleague wanting to let me know that she and her husband were expecting a baby girl. I was unbelievably distraught, I knew that this would happen, I just wished it didn't have to happen so soon. The fact it was a baby girl seemed to make me even more upset.

Everyone else was experiencing such exciting milestones in life and I was trying to learn to adapt to my new normal, a life I hadn't planned or wanted.

A week after that text message I received another message from a good friend who had looked up the best way to tell me her news. She was pregnant with her second baby.

My heart hurt so much for so many reasons. I was happy for everyone who shared this news with me, but I was unbelievably sad for myself and my family. I was sad because our babies would never get to meet and about the future they would never get to share.

It took me almost two months to feel ready to be able to go out for dinner with my girlfriends. They had all visited me individually, but it was my first time actually being out in a group and I was so incredibly nervous.

I asked Chris before we went what I was supposed to talk about. I felt like I had nothing in common with them anymore and didn't want to dampen their happiness.

Out of the four of them, one was recently married, one had just had her third baby and the other two were pregnant with their second babies. Their lives were moving forward in an incredibly exciting direction and I was waiting for autopsy results to find out if Chris and I would even be able to have children together.

I was sitting at the table listening to everyone discuss the inevitable topic of children. The children people had, the ones they were expecting and who may join the club next. You know the conversation! I'm sure you've had it countless times, especially if you're over the age of twenty-eight.

Well, you never know the backstories of everyone on the edge of these discussions, or the pain they might be hiding. I'm not saying this to make you feel guilty but because it's the truth, with so many couples, and singles, experiencing infertility and the loss of babies.

I remember plastering the smile on my face, feeling the fuzzy feeling in my nose. The one that happens when you really fight the intense need to cry. I hoped with all my heart I wasn't addressed in the conversation as I knew as soon as I opened my mouth the tears would fall. And once asked a question, they did.

I couldn't stop them. In the middle of the restaurant, I cried.

I cried because I couldn't help it and because my life was now so different to all of theirs. I cried because I didn't know if I would ever have any living children of my own. I cried because my heart was broken and there was nothing anyone could say or do to make it better.

Facebook and Instagram were and continue to be an absolute minefield for me. They became more like 'Babybook' and 'Babygram'. They have both been incredible tools in my healing journey and have helped me learn so much and connect with so many people who have experienced similar losses. But they have also made me feel completely devastated.

As a thirty-year-old female, I see a lot of baby photos and pregnancy announcements in my feed. In the first few months after having Violet there were at least five pregnancy announcements and two birth announcements from various acquaintances and old work colleagues.

Strangely for me, it was never the general photos people posted of their babies or children that really upset me, it was the weekly and monthly updates. Before losing Violet, I used to think they were absolutely adorable and loved seeing how much my friends' babies had grown, but now they left me feeling broken.

In my head when I would see a post that said, *Three months old today!* I would calculate the months it had been since I had Violet or how old she would be if she were born on her due date. For quite a few months whilst I was in this state, I had to mute many good friends so I could avoid looking at their pictures.

As the months progressed, so did everyone else's lives. My phone rang far less and I was no longer receiving daily text messages asking how I was. I began to make more of an effort to connect with my close friends and started asking them how they were and what was going on in their lives.

It was nice to be distracted and hear what was going on in other people's lives (as long as it wasn't baby related, of course) but it was also a painful reminder that the world keeps moving on even if I wasn't ready to.

Within the first six months since Violet died, I had six people close to me let me know that they were pregnant.

One day, a family member asked me to pop around to her house after work, I hadn't spoken to her much recently so thought it would be a good chance to catch up. I had no idea what was coming.

When I walked into her house, she was really awkward and instantly I could tell she had to get something off her chest.

'I've got something to tell you,' she said. 'We're having a baby and I didn't want you to find out when we announced it on Facebook. It wasn't planned at all, but we are really excited.'

I knew she thought she was doing a good thing in giving me advance warning, but in that moment I was upset and angry with her: How did she expect me to react? Didn't she know how much pressure it put on me, calling me on a 'date' and telling me to my face. If I'd learnt through a text message, or even through the internet, I'd have time to process my mixed emotions—and hide them from her.

I can't even remember exactly what my response was. I know it wasn't congratulations and I know that I didn't give her the level of excitement she wanted or deserved. It felt like a punch in the stomach and I'm pretty sure I acted that way.

I told another friend that I will forever be grateful to those who messaged me first. This surprised her and she said she thought it would be nicer and more considerate face-to-face. My reason for that is those who messaged me gave me the opportunity to react in my own way before I pulled myself together and congratulated them; by the time I saw each person

I was excitedly asking questions and celebrating in their joy.

I know that I didn't react in the way that my family member who told me to my face had hoped, I felt sick about it all that night and sent an apology message for my response. She was also clearly disappointed that I wasn't as initially excited as she had hoped.

I also know another friend who had lost a baby and had been through multiple failed cycles of IVF who was taken out to lunch by her cousin, who shared that she was pregnant. I can't imagine how difficult that would have been, my friend had to sit in a restaurant with no escape and act happy for the next hour or so. She then got in her car and hysterically cried until she was ready to drive herself home.

The honest truth is, when someone has recently lost a baby or is struggling to conceive a child of their own, the announcement of someone else's pregnancy is hard for so many reasons. But the reason is never because they are unhappy for you. It is because it is another reminder of something that they don't have but desperately want, it is because they wish your kids could be friends, it is because they can't understand why it was easy for you to fall pregnant and they have spent thousands of dollars on IVF with no success, it is because when you show them an ultrasound image they are remembering what it felt like at the ultrasound clinic to be told that their baby didn't have a heartbeat.

One of my beautiful friends wrote in her text message: 'I am telling you this way so you can be mad or sad or do whatever it is you need to do and then you can respond when you are ready.' I am so thankful to her and everyone else who messaged as it gave me a moment to breathe and compose the response I wanted to give.

In the early days after my loss and return to work I also asked my bosses to either share pregnancy announcements in advance or to let me know if there was going to be one made. This helped ensure that my initial reaction wasn't in front of a group of people.

I found that often once the announcement was made, people would scan the room to find my face and see how I was. Sometimes out of kindness and concern and other times out of curiosity.

About six months into my grieving journey a close friend confided face-to-face she was pregnant and I didn't instantly burst into tears or say the wrong thing. I asked questions and we spoke about how she was feeling. About five minutes into our conversation she asked if I was okay as she could see my eyes getting watery. We later discussed how hard I found it finding out face-to-face and she felt awful.

It was then I realised how important it was for her and probably others to be able to share their exciting news face-to-face. I even remembered when I first found out I was pregnant and made sure I told everyone to their face as it felt more special.

As time has moved on, I have still felt impacted by pregnancy and baby announcements, but I have been able to bounce back quicker.

In the initial few months, I would find hearing about a friend's pregnancy could seriously impact my mood and mental state for a good few days. When I hear about it now, I feel a little bit sad, but it doesn't take as long to move forward and doesn't have as much of a lingering impact.

I have also been able to hold babies without feeling like my heart would break. This is something for a while there I genuinely couldn't imagine being able to do.

I remember at support group hearing a lady share how she had held her best friend's baby only one month after losing her own and I couldn't actually understand how she had managed to do it without falling apart in the process.

The first baby I held was born on the day I found out Violet wasn't well or going to be okay. I didn't see him when he was born, it actually took me five months before I felt ready to see him and when I did it was beautiful. He was no longer a newborn baby and was easy to hold. He nuzzled into my neck with a cuddle and it felt unbelievably healing.

One of my best friends gave birth six months after saying goodbye to Violet. When she confided in me that she was pregnant I was about fourteen weeks and although we didn't know if things were okay with my baby, we fantasised about how nice it would be to go through our pregnancies together and how beautiful it would be to have our babies so close in age.

The loss of Violet greatly impacted her. I know each step of her pregnancy was often a hard reminder of what I no longer had or was going to experience.

Her beautiful baby girl arrived at the beginning of the new year absolutely perfect. I had decided not to visit at the hospital as I felt it may have been too much, but I was there as soon as she returned home. Chris and I drove there with our home-cooked meal and presents, apprehensive about how we would feel once we arrived.

As soon as I saw her beautiful baby, my apprehension disappeared. She was absolutely divine and didn't at all trigger me or remind me of Violet. I realised holding her that no baby will ever remind me of Violet as no baby will ever be the same as her.

Holding my friend's gorgeous five-day-old baby was comforting and reminded me how miraculous pregnancy and birth is.

When discussing her birth experience, I was able to relate and share elements of mine and that was an important part in it being okay. I think if we had met her baby girl with the intention of pretending mine didn't exist it would have been a completely different experience.

The surprise pregnancy announcement party just before Christmas and New Year's Eve provided big steps forward for me. Leading up to New Year's Eve my social media feed was full of bereaved mums sharing how upset they were to be heading into the new year as it would be another year that their baby didn't exist. For those who had lost their baby that year, they didn't want to welcome or celebrate New Year's Eve as they felt it was another step forward in leaving their baby behind.

Prior to reading this on social media the thought had honestly not occurred to me, but once it was placed in my mind I couldn't get it out. I began feeling upset and anxious about celebrating, it began to feel like in celebrating New Year's Eve I was celebrating moving away from my baby girl.

I also had a few people say to me leading up to the new year that they hoped my 2020 was better as they couldn't imagine it could be much worse than 2019. I had one person describe 2019 as the worst year they could have imagined for me, and others use words like awful and horrible to describe it. This also didn't sit well for me, because although 2019 was a challenging year, it was also amazing. It was the year I became a mum and the year my beautiful baby girl entered into the world.

We were invited to a New Year's Eve party and like with all things I had said we may or may not attend depending on how we felt on the day. The day came around and I decided it was the perfect time to declutter and clean out our house.

During the therapeutic motions of decluttering our house I realised that one calendar day doesn't change how I feel about Violet, it doesn't mean I am moving further away from her as she is always with me in everything I do.

At the very last minute I decided to go to the party and it was a really nice night. We were able to celebrate with everyone else knowing that our girl is a part of all we do and we are taking her with us wherever we go moving forward.

New Year's Eve was the first time I had a celebratory drink of alcohol since January.

It took me five months before I considered eating soft cheeses (something I have always loved) as during pregnancy it is one of the biggest no-noes and it was something I envisioned eating as a celebration in the hospital room with some champagne. Many of my friends had turned up to the hospital to meet one another's babies with a little pack of goodies that you couldn't have during pregnancy, things like soft cheeses, deli meats and alcohol. That's how I thought my experience was going to go and I was sad, yet another moment that was taken away from me.

Having a drink on New Year's Eve was a big deal—although nobody celebrating with us would have guessed. As I took that first sip of wine, I realised that it was okay to be happy and to celebrate and have fun. That doing those things didn't move me further away from Violet and they didn't mean I loved her any less.

Although my life is in limbo in regard to further expanding our family and having children, I found that when I was ready it was important for me that I wasn't in limbo in other areas. Having other interests and focuses has been such an important part in coping with each and every pregnancy announcement and birth for me.

It took me at least five months and ten chapters to feel brave enough to share with people that I was writing a book. I'm not sure if they all believed me, but it has been a great focus for me and provided an interesting conversation topic.

When I felt ready, I also began focusing a lot of energy on my career and applying for various opportunities and roles, something I know wouldn't have been possible if I had a newborn baby. Just over six months after losing Violet I got an exciting new job that twelve months earlier I couldn't have dreamed of.

When I got my new job, I was so excited about it but also had mixed feelings and emotions. Although I know it wouldn't have been possible if Violet were here, I tried to focus on celebrating that she is the reason it was possible. She gave me the strength and courage to apply and put myself out there.

Violet's Gift has also helped ensure that I am working towards something and not just waiting as time moves forward. I currently have more interests and hobbies than I ever have before, and my life feels less in limbo. I am able to join in again. I just have a different perspective and I no longer do things because it is right or because I have to. I do things because I enjoy them—and I want to.

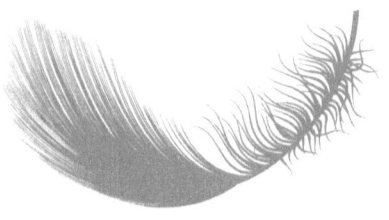

*When someone has recently lost a baby or is struggling to conceive a child of their own, the announcement of someone else's pregnancy is hard for so many reasons. But the reason is never because they are unhappy for you.*

## CHAPTER ELEVEN
# Remembering Violet

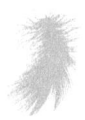

In the doorway of the function room I placed a chalk board to welcome friends and family members with the greeting: *Welcome to Violet's Celebration.* As I chalked the letters onto the sign underneath a string of rainbow pompoms, I thought, for the thousandth time since her death, how surreal our life had become since then. And how resilient humans really can be.

It was only five weeks after Violet was born that we selected a date that worked for us and our families and began preparations for what we called a 'Celebration of Violet'. At the time, I knew that—in the future—we'd want and need to do something to commemorate her, even if we weren't ready to hold a 'celebration' yet.

If people didn't understand, we would explain it was a memorial. At the time, we sent a save-the-date text to everyone we wanted to invite and explained that we had chosen the day to celebrate our beautiful baby girl and all of the love she has brought into our lives. We explained that we had never done anything like this before or been to something like this, so were just working it out as we went along.

It was here. The date we'd chosen what felt like a lifetime

ago. I needed to find the courage to celebrate our little girl's life—because she deserved it, and so did we.

When you lose a baby, you aren't just losing a newborn. You are losing your toddler taking their first step. Your child's first day of school. Your teenager getting their first job. Your adult child getting married.

You lose every magical moment when you lose a child.

I think it only took one month before I started to forget what it felt like to hold Violet in my arms. I spent so much time looking at her photos, trying to conjure the physical feeling of being together. I felt so disconnected from her and it hurt my heart.

The feeling reminded me of when you come back from a big holiday and very quickly it feels like you never went. Or after your wedding day, you know it was the best day ever and you love looking at the photos, but you don't feel as connected to it.

Life goes on and that feeling of not remembering so well and leaving Violet behind made me feel so incredibly guilty and sad.

How would you feel forgetting what it felt like to hold your baby and not getting another chance? How would you move forward with your life knowing that your baby would never get to move forward with theirs?

I know with all my heart that I will never forget Violet, she will always be with me and will always be my first baby. She is the one who made me a mum and Chris a dad and she has completely changed us as people.

It has been extremely important for me to keep Violet's memory alive and to help make her mark on the world.

I am a parent but being a parent has looked very different for me. It hasn't involved researching the best prams or nappies and I haven't been inundated with advice nor have I been handed a parenting book to help me navigate. Like everyone else who has walked this challenging path of parenthood, I have worked it out along the way.

I have experienced a different kind of parenthood.

Creating Violet's memory began when we chose her name. As I have mentioned, when we knew we were most likely going to be saying goodbye to our baby, the names we had on our list no longer felt right. We needed a name with meaning. I have always been a fan of floral names and when I read the meaning of the name Violet to Chris, he cried and said that's the one.

According to various sources, the colour violet is said to assist those who seek the meaning of life and spiritual fulfillment. It is also associated with transformation of the soul and a link between spiritual and physical worlds. The colour violet is meant to inspire unconditional and selfless love and knowing this, we believe we couldn't have found a more fitting name for our beautiful daughter whom we love so much.

We also love that violet is the last colour in a rainbow, and we would have beautiful violet flowers to always remember her by.

We chose the name Grace as a middle name as it sounds great with Violet and means beauty, kindness and thanks.

When we returned from hospital, we received so many beautiful violet-coloured flowers and gifts. Both of my nannas picked and pressed violet flowers from their gardens on the day she was born. Each time our close family and friends see rainbows they send us pictures of them and let us know that they are thinking of our girl. Some people even just send me text messages with the rainbow and purple heart emoji. I have also received messages from those not so close to us about violet flowers they have seen that reminded them of our baby.

Seeing rainbows and violet flowers help us feel connected to our girl.

The first day Chris returned to work I went to Bunnings and spent an hour selecting the perfect violet flowers. I came home and immediately potted the flowers in two large pots in our front yard, so every time we go out and come home again they are often the first thing we see.

There isn't only guilt about what you do—but also what you don't.

On Facebook pages for bereaved parents, or at our support group, whenever I'd hear that another bereaved parent had done something for their baby that I hadn't done, like set up a memorial space in their house or get a tattoo of their baby's name, I'd question myself. *Should we be doing that too? Should we be doing more?*

I believe that how we chose to honour Violet is completely unique to me and my family. It is not necessarily what another family who have lost a baby would do. Everyone parents in their own way and honours their baby's memory in the way that works for them.

How would you stay connected to a baby that is no longer here?

Over time, I'd developed a rule that worked for me. If I kept thinking about something repeatedly that I wasn't sure if I wanted to do for her then I just had to do it. This rule helped ensure that I didn't have regrets.

At times, doing what I wanted to do or thought of may have also meant ignoring the comments of well-meaning family members who thought certain things may not be necessary (like having a photographer at her memorial, no regrets!). This has actually been a great life lesson for me with so many things.

One of my biggest acts in remembering Violet was to record and write our story (some of which you are currently reading).

As I have mentioned, in the first few days after returning from the hospital I was absolutely terrified that I would forget the smaller details of my pregnancy and Violet's birth. I would sit at my laptop for hours, often forgetting to take a break. I cried constantly as my fingers connected with the keyboard and pages and pages of words took form. I felt as if I were telling someone else's story. I wasn't writing for an audience, and I wasn't writing with the intention of creating a book or even showing anyone, I was just writing a chronological recount of what we had been through to ensure no detail was missed.

Continuing to write our story has been a beautiful way for me to stay connected with Violet and to not feel like I am just moving on. I would spend days at work surrounded by people who never mentioned Violet and would look forward to coming home so I could continue to work on our story and remain connected.

I know many people who have created an altar or shrine for their baby or other lost loved one. But I decided early on that this was not what I wanted, I wanted to include Violet in our home like I would have if she were alive. I printed and framed photos of her and included them in our photo wall surrounded by wedding photos, which is where her baby photos would have been. We have photos of her in our bedroom and her urn is on a shelf in our living area surrounded by crystals, plants and art.

After spending the first month on our dining room table, her belongings from the hospital have been placed in a personalised keepsake box. Chris and I also carry a part of her with us each day in our jewellery that we wear.

The thought of having a funeral or memorial straight after Violet was born was far too much for our minds to comprehend. We had made so many difficult decisions and organised so many challenging things that we just couldn't do it.

I think having a funeral at that time would have completely broken me, I genuinely don't know if I could have emotionally survived it. In saying that, we also knew that we wanted to eventually do something to honour our baby girl when we felt ready.

In the week leading up to Violet's Celebration I was so excited to finally have the opportunity to celebrate her in a way she deserved. I kept myself busy preparing all of the small details as I knew that this was the only big celebration she would get and it needed to be just right.

The day of the celebration couldn't have been more perfect. It was held eleven weeks after we welcomed Violet into the world and it gave us enough time to have everything exactly as we wanted.

We held it at a function room at our local lifesaving club overlooking the ocean. We requested no children and made the decision to only invite those closest to us who had been there for us throughout the pregnancy, Violet's birth and the weeks that followed. We organised beautiful invitations that were designed by the same talented lady who made our wedding invitations and had well-thought-out decorations, small touches and menus.

The day before Violet's celebration I felt really excited to have the opportunity to actually celebrate our beautiful girl. The theme was rainbow and violet.

Chris made rainbow cupcakes, which was our first attempt at icing cupcakes and was far more difficult than the YouTube videos made out. Our sweet menu also had fairy bread, rainbow fruit sticks, violet crumble slice and sugar cookies with violet-coloured icing and the word 'love' stamped on them, as well as chocolate digestives as they were a go-to pregnancy food.

We spent the day before finalising the food and decorations and creating jars of violet-coloured flowers to place around the room. The mood was uplifting, we both felt happy we were able to do this for our girl.

As I lay in bed that night, the excitement that I had felt earlier had completely disappeared and in the silence of our room my tears poured. I should have been thirty-four weeks pregnant and having a baby shower in anticipation of welcoming my baby. I shouldn't have been running through the words I was going to say at a memorial for my baby. It felt so unbelievably unfair.

When I woke up in the morning, I could feel the adrenaline pulsing through my body. I was so on edge and just wanted everything to be absolutely perfect for our girl.

We got ready and packed the car full of everything we had prepared and made our way to the lifesaving club. We were met there by my family and began the set up.

I was a little bit like a drill sergeant directing everyone to what I needed them to do. I recall myself saying at one stage, 'Is there anyone who doesn't have a job at the moment? Because I've got a list.' Everything was perfect and ready quicker than I had anticipated. I remember standing there enjoying the view and feeling impressed by our efforts with how good everything looked.

It wasn't until the first person arrived that the wave of emotions hit me. In the set up, I had almost distracted myself from the reason we were all there. I cried as I greeted each loving friend and family member. This was probably the first time a lot of them had seen me completely and utterly vulnerable in my heartbreak. I had held it together in front of most people and had become skilled at removing my emotions when telling our story, but today wasn't the day to hold anything together.

There were lots of tears (not just from me), but also smiles and laughs as people read the little signs I had placed around the room.

I had placed signs saying:

*Violet's favourite food*

*Did you know Meagan ate 1–2 packets of chocolate digestives a week when pregnant?*

*Violet loved them*

*Her other favourite foods include oranges, pancakes, Time Out chocolate bars and KFC Popcorn Chicken Go Buckets (she takes after her daddy)*

I had other signs sharing her favourite music based on how much she had danced around when we placed headphones on my stomach and played different songs for her.

We had photos displayed of our ultrasounds, bump photos and photos of Violet and us as a family from when we were in hospital. We had a sign with her birth details and most importantly had her urn with a candle burning.

Only our immediate family had met Violet in hospital and a lot of people remarked on the day that they felt they were meeting her for the first time. Those who didn't fully grasp or comprehend our loss could now understand.

One person who had said we would eventually get over it once we had another baby was completely distraught and apologised profusely for their insensitive comment. They just hadn't understood.

To include everyone in the day, we gave out little candles bearing Violet's name and birthdate as well as the quote: *Let this light shine up above and wrap you tight in all our love.* We asked everyone there to light the candle on Violet's due date and birth date and send us a photo.

We know that each person there would have done anything they could to take away some of our pain, but unfortunately no one could change what had happened or bring our baby back. In lighting a candle and sending us a photo on those days, it helped us know how loved our baby and we were. It also gave everyone in the room something that they could do to help us.

Once they had arrived, everyone stood around in the room unsure of what to expect or what the proceedings would be. Chris and I began by each saying a few words. We thanked everyone for their love and support and acknowledged how challenging our journey into parenthood had been. We shared how meeting Violet for the first time was the best moment of our lives and how much love we have for our girl.

We followed this by listening to the beautiful song 'Winter Bear' by Coby Grant. I discovered this song only a number of days after Violet was born and I still can't listen to it without turning into a blubbering mess. I felt the song was almost written about our beautiful girl; she was born in winter and some of the lyrics are *I love you to the moon and back,* which is what I wrote in a book we read to Violet in hospital.

During this stage of the day boxes of tissues were being handed around as I don't think there was a dry eye in the room.

Once we had listened to the first few verses in the song, we all walked out onto the decking overlooking the ocean. We had purchased purple bubble wands and attached the words *A tiny life so brief and small, the love you gave has changed us all.* No one spoke as we all stood there and blew bubbles with our thoughts and love for Violet.

The love felt on the decking was incredibly moving. The water was perfectly still, the sun shone out from behind the clouds. I wasn't the only person who knew we were being watched over by the girl we were all celebrating.

We were all completely and utterly exhausted from the emotions and returned to the room to eat some of the delicious food and mingle. Those who hadn't read the signs or enjoyed the decorations and photos earlier walked around and got to know Violet.

We had the beautiful book *Born to Fly* by Tamara J. Whittaker on display and we asked everyone there on the day to write a message to Violet on the blank pages at the front and back of the book.

Before I knew it, the day was over and we were hugging everyone goodbye. Once we had packed up, Chris and I sat on the pier and reflected on what a perfect day we had celebrating our unbelievably perfect girl. We discussed how perfect every detail was and how emotional we had felt. We also discussed how it didn't feel like goodbye or closure and we were glad for that. We didn't want to say goodbye.

The morning after, I felt like I had an emotional hangover—but no regrets. I could already tell the celebration had been cathartic, for me anyway. This was the first time I really started to think about how we would move forward without our baby in our lives.

I was returning to work from my maternity leave the following day and knew that thinking about Violet and doing things to connect me to her was no longer going to take up all of my days. It was time for me to re-enter the world and I felt ready.

Four weeks after I had given birth and Chris had returned to work, I parked my car in the carpark and walked back into the hospital—the scene of so much trauma and heartbreak. I had a meeting scheduled with the social worker and head of the women's health unit of the hospital where Violet was born.

My stomach did turn in knots when I walked through the door, but I was there with a purpose and a renewed passion to do something positive.

We had a lot of family, friends and colleagues express that they would like to make a donation in memory of Violet but would like us to indicate whom to donate to. Chris and I spent a lot of time thinking about this, but nothing felt quite right. We decided that we wanted to do all we could to keep Violet's memory alive and make a difference for parents that find themselves in a situation similar to ours.

During my maternity leave, I had gone through all the paperwork I had left the hospital with and tried to find a phone number for someone I could call to ask about making a donation in memory of Violet. We had some ideas but didn't want to donate just anything to the hospital, especially if they didn't have a need for it.

I eventually found the phone number of the social worker and contacted her with our idea—which she liked!

In addition to discussing making a donation, they asked if I would be willing to provide feedback on my experience. The social worker met me in the foyer, we walked into the maternity ward together.

I had dressed like I was going to a meeting for work, I had properly dried and straightened my hair and put on makeup for the first time in a couple of months. I looked like a very different person to how I was at our last meeting, so much so that the social worker actually didn't recognise me.

I had zero expectations about this meeting, I was hoping my feedback might be of use but I was mainly hoping to organise to do something small in Violet's memory. The meeting lasted two hours and was so much more than I could have hoped for. As I provided feedback, both women took notes and discussed possible changes that could be made. I shared how traumatic it was to sit in the waiting room with other pregnant women when I was about to say goodbye to my baby and this was something that they said they could change immediately.

Once we finished discussing my experience at the hospital, we moved on to talking about making a donation in Violet's memory. I shared my basic ideas of maybe a Cuddle Cot or something and I asked them if they had any ideas or anything they needed.

The conversation was exciting and fruitful. I left with a notebook full of ideas and we all had various action items.

That night I shared the meeting details with Chris. We decided to try and achieve all of the ideas I had written down in my notebook.

We decided to create a fundraising campaign that would allow us to purchase and donate the various items and resources to the hospital to help support other grieving families who found themselves in a similar situation to us.

Once I had received the quotes from the team at the hospital I began working on the campaign. I met with a friend and her daughter who specialises in social media and communications. In that meeting I learnt what a content calendar is and came up with a plan on how I was going to fundraise and get the message out there.

There was just one thing I still didn't have and that was a name.

They asked me to clarify what my goal was and I explained I wanted to gift items to the hospital that would help grieving families in Violet's memory. This is how Violet's Gift was born—but I didn't realise at that point what it would become!

It's amazing how, when you really create something with love and it's meant to be, it all happens so quickly. In a matter of weeks—with the help of many kind friends with different skills—we had a logo, a content calendar for social media and all the promotional content ready to go!

I couldn't believe how fast it was happening!

On the week of Violet's due date, I met with the hospital to confirm our plans for fundraising to ensure we were following all of the guidelines. I contacted family and friends to get them involved in sharing our message and various pages. I had set up a GoFundMe page where people could donate and a Facebook page that shared more information about our journey.

If we could meet our goal of $8,000, we would be able to create a special room where grieving parents could recover from childbirth and spend precious time with their baby in a warm and non-sterile hospital environment.

If we could meet our target of $10,000, we would be able to create the special room plus a memory tree that would go in the sacred space at the hospital. This tree would have the names of the babies lost at the hospital placed on the leaves, a place where families could go and remember the babies who were gone too soon.

If we could meet our target of $15,000, we would be able to create the special room and the memory tree and purchase a portable Cuddle Cot for the hospital (a system that allows for babies who have passed away to remain with their families in their home so that they are not required to be cooled in a mortuary environment).

And, if we surpassed those targets, any additional money raised would be donated to Heartfelt, a volunteer organisation of professional photographers from all over Australia and New Zealand dedicated to giving the gift of photographic memories to families that have experienced stillbirths or premature births or have children with serious and terminal illnesses.

On Violet's due date, 15 November, we launched Violet's Gift into the public space, with an announcement on Facebook:

> Today is Violet's due date.
>
> To honour our beautiful girl, we are excited to launch 'Violet's Gift', a way for us to keep our daughter's memory alive and to make a difference

to local parents and families that find themselves in a situation similar to ours.

To be able to make the difference we would like, we need your support. Please consider sharing Violet's Gift with others in your life. If you would like to make a donation to help us support families who experience the loss of a baby head to the link below.

Our plan was to post about Violet's Gift on our social media accounts and not look at any of it again until the Sunday. We had organised to get away and go to the beach for the weekend with our puppies and spend Violet's due date together as a family.

We got up early and shed a couple of tears at the reality of our situation. We wished that instead of launching a campaign to raise money we were instead being woken up throughout the night by a crying baby or potentially awaiting the arrival of our beautiful baby.

We had a beautiful and relaxing day together. Our willpower to not check our GoFundMe page wasn't very strong, that afternoon we looked and had already raised almost $5,000. We were so overwhelmed by the kindness and love we were receiving.

Over the weekend the donations had continued and within the first week we had raised almost $10,000. The messages we were receiving were so incredibly touching. So many people I had never met were reaching out to thank us for sharing our experience. I had more than one mum contact me to share their experiences of loss and that they wished that all of this had been available to them.

I had one loss mama thank me for providing her with the opportunity to make a donation in memory of her baby. She shared that she hadn't had the strength during and immediately after her loss to thank those who had made a difference to her experience and she felt this was her way.

One of our Facebook posts sharing our experience of loss received over 10,000 views and knowing that we were helping people with their own experiences just through sharing ours meant so much to me.

So many people helped share our fundraiser, we even had a friend raise money for Violet's Gift by shaving his head. In one month of launching Violet's Gift, we raised almost $12,000, started numerous conversations and people were talking about baby loss and pregnancy loss.

To help us reach our final fundraising target, we contacted some small businesses to see if they would consider collaborating with us. We had people who sold candles donate a small profit, one lady who created beautiful lanyards and key rings made a specific Violet's Gift lanyard and key ring to help raise money. Another generous woman who creates stylish and practical accessories for little ones reached out to a graphic designer and designed a range of special bibs in collaboration with Violet's Gift.

It took just over three months for us to exceed our

fundraising target, but Violet's Gift became so much bigger than just fundraising.

Five weeks after launching Violet's Gift a message I'll never forget dropped into my Instagram inbox. It read:

> Hi Meagan, my name is Kate, and I gave birth to my daughter in March this year at the same hospital you had Violet. She was born at thirty weeks gestation. I just saw your fundraiser and I think it's a beautiful idea. I wish I had somewhere I could have taken our daughter to spend some time rather than just the hospital room. I'm so touched by what you are doing and would love to offer any help I can. I am donating now in hope that other families can spend enough precious time with their babies because they have to also walk out of the door empty handed. Sending so much love mumma, Violet would be so proud to have you as her mum xxx

When I launched Violet's Gift, I thought I did it to keep our daughter's memory alive, and to support other parents going through what we had experienced. But quickly I was realising this could be a lifeline to me too.

It felt so important to me that we develop new traditions where Violet is included. For Christmas, I purchased a personalised ornament with Violet's name on it. That way she would be with us no matter where we had Christmas.

When we took our standard family photos on Christmas Day, I held the personalised ornament with Violet's name on it. I look at those photos and feel so many mixed emotions. It is hard to believe that we should have been holding a one-month-old baby, not a Christmas ornament.

One week before Christmas we went to the shops to buy gifts for Violet. We decided that we still wanted the opportunity to do that, but instead of taking them home and wrapping them or putting them in a stocking for Christmas morning, we donated them to a local charity.

On Christmas Day, as my social media feed filled up with family photographs, I wanted to acknowledge our family, in its entirety. I created a cartoon, using a free computer program, that showed Chris and me, Violet and our two dogs, Charlie and Tilly, together.

I posted it on our social media accounts with the caption: *Merry Christmas from our family to yours. Sending lots of love and strength to those with someone missing today. May your grief and joy co-exist and may you hear your loved one's name said aloud.*

We received lots of responses from friends and family. Everyone wished us a Merry Christmas in return and many people commented how beautiful the photo was.

For me, it was just special to be able to share a photo of my family on a significant day. It might not have been as I had planned or looked like any of the photos my friends posted. But it was perfect for us.

*When you lose a baby, you aren't just losing a newborn. You are losing your toddler taking their first step. Your child's first day of school. Your teenager getting their first job. Your adult child getting married. You lose every magical moment when you lose a child.*

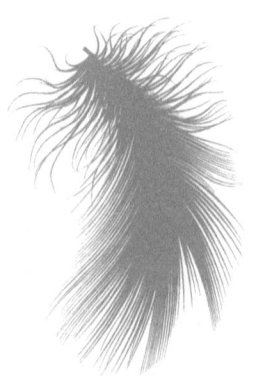

## CHAPTER TWELVE
# Why me, what next?

At our first support group meeting one of the most prominent comments and discussion topics was *Why me?* The other people in the group were asking why this had to happen to them. One mum wondered if it was because she slept on the wrong side whilst another questioned if it was because of something she ate.

All anyone wanted was answers about why this had to happen to them. Why were we the ones sitting in a community centre room crying about the loss of our babies when other mums would be in the same space the next day enjoying their first mothers group.

I have learnt through this community that, sadly, many people are left with no answers about why their baby's heart stopped beating, which often leaves them with more and more questions.

I know a friend's mum who had a stillborn baby over thirty years ago who still wonders if it happened because she smoked in the lead-up to her pregnancy.

Our story was obviously different again as I never had any questions about why Violet's heart stopped beating. I never wondered if it was something I did … because I knew. I knew that Violet was incredibly unwell, and it seemed that the reason was Chris and I appeared to both be carriers of the same gene mutation. This isn't something you think to ask each other on your first date!

During our very first meeting with the geneticist after finding out about Violet's condition, I tried my best to understand the science—a subject that has never been my forte. One of the questions they asked us during that meeting was: 'Is there any chance the two of you could be related?' I felt shocked and embarrassed and remembered very clearly thinking that they were trying to politely tell us that we weren't actually compatible.

After clarifying that we definitely weren't related and asking if we weren't compatible, I was kindly reassured that wasn't the case, but having future children wouldn't be straightforward for us.

In that appointment I learnt that each person is a carrier of some gene mutations, often we live our lives not knowing as it doesn't really affect us.

If it was confirmed that, yes, Chris and I were both carriers of the same gene mutation, then statistics and science would indicate a one in four chance that what occurred in Violet would happen again.

Over time, you begin to move from *Why me?* to another question:

What next?

And, there isn't always a simple answer.

It is assumed by so many people when you lose a baby that

you will immediately start trying again. I remember my first week back at work and a colleague asked me when we thought we would try again.

I also know of many people where this is the case.

In the online forums and Facebook groups, one of the most common questions people ask is when you can start trying again or when it is safe to do so. Some women even mention that they felt focusing on having another baby was an important part of their healing.

Our options for having children aren't as simple as waiting until it's safe. They involve a lot of waiting for medical appointments and reliance on modern medicine.

In our first genetics appointment, just after Violet's due date, we were told we could try naturally to conceive and the doctors would be able to do tests at twelve to thirteen weeks gestation to identify if our baby was healthy.

The risk? It could all happen again!

As soon as we heard this, Chris and I both agreed without hesitation this was not an option for us. We could not go through what we were currently going through a second time. The thought of it was unbearable.

So, what are the other options for us?

I have since met and spoken to three different people who made the decision to 'just try again'. They decided that they wanted a healthy baby so badly that they would continue trying until they got it. All of their reasons were different and I have absolutely no judgement. In fact, I admire their strength.

One woman I had spoken to had made this decision with her

husband because of the cost of IVF and embryo testing, at this stage she has had to end two pregnancies and does not have a healthy baby in her arms. Another couple, who we met through our support group, ended three pregnancies because each baby was incredibly sick, but they were determined to keep trying until they had a healthy baby. They didn't want to have to wait for the results of further research and embryo testing.

Each of the people who had made the decision to keep trying naturally were in their late thirties and concerned about how much time they had left.

When Violet was born, I was thirty and Chris was thirty-two. So, we decided to undergo the genetic tests to try and find an answer, because we had a little more time on our side. We had also decided to go ahead with an autopsy knowing it could take up to twelve months to get the results.

We were used to waiting games by this point.

I know lots of people who chose not to do an autopsy as they can't imagine putting their baby through that and I can completely understand. The thought of it is absolutely horrific. But I also know how important it was for us.

Without Violet's diagnosis and DNA, we have no chance at doing IVF and providing her with siblings.

Three days after Violet's due date and the launch of Violet's Gift I received a phone call with the information that our autopsy results were ready.

A few days later, at the hospital—the same place where we last heard Violet's heartbeat—we received the news: the doctor's earlier prognosis was right, and their suspected diagnosis matched the autopsy results.

So, now we had answers to the question: Why us?

So, what next?

It was six months since Violet's passing when we received a phone call letting us know that they had identified the gene that had caused her condition. We also discovered that Chris and I are confirmed carriers. It might sound odd, but I felt such a wave of relief and happiness for knowing something was certain.

When the phone call came, I said to our specialist, 'This is good news, isn't it?'

She responded, 'We don't use the word *good*, we use the word *hopeful*.'

At least this meant that we had a plan and could begin the process of seeing if we were eligible for IVF.

If we were fortunate enough to go through the IVF process and pre-implantation diagnosis to fall pregnant, we would still go through the 'normal' uncertainties of pregnancy, anxiously awaiting the testing and scans, hoping with all our hearts that our baby is healthy and okay.

As I write this, we have had an initial meeting with an IVF specialist, we have undertaken the various blood tests and scans to see if it is possible for us to go down this path. We have completed our National Police Checks (who knew that was a thing for IVF!) and we have another appointment scheduled in five weeks where we will hopefully have more answers and direction.

I know that the path of IVF is not an easy one to travel. I know that it can be heartbreaking and challenging. I have read that to do IVF you need three things: time, money and strength. At this stage we have all three, but we also know that it is only the beginning.

It is important for me not to wait to finish this book with a hopeful 'fairytale ending' where I announce to everyone that we had another baby and all lived happily ever after.

In the beginning stages of my loss and grief they were my least favourite stories to hear. It seemed everyone I connected with who had also experienced pregnancy loss was now happily in the next stage of their life with a bundle of joy and it absolutely devastated me. I wanted to hear from those who still had big question marks about the next stage.

I have no idea if that will be my story and I don't know for certain if I will be fortunate enough to have other children.

Because Violet is my first child, I know that I have lost the opportunity to ever have a positive, carefree pregnancy experience. However, because of her I am much more resilient than I ever thought possible. I know that no matter the outcome I will be okay.

I have been warned by many health experts that pregnancy after loss can be traumatic and have a huge toll on my mental health. However, my experience has made me truly appreciate what a miracle pregnancy and birth is. I know that there will be many challenges but also so much to celebrate too.

We still don't know what the future holds for us and our family, but whatever happens, I know that we are going to be okay!

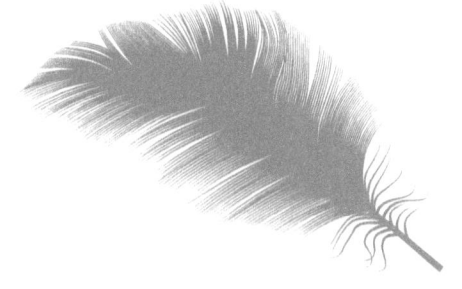

*Over time, you begin to move from Why us?*
*to another question:*
*What next?*
*And there isn't always a simple answer.*

CHAPTER THIRTEEN
# Everything I wish I knew

The winter that Violet was born was over, I got through the spring in a blur, summer came and went, and on the year flew. Somewhere along the way, I realised that my role had changed (again!). I was moving from victim to survivor—from broken to overcoming—from the person who needed to be helped to a helper.

'We've had a miscarriage.' When I saw the message from my friend's husband, my heart broke for her instantly.

Anna was eighteen weeks pregnant with a very wanted baby that they had tried for over four years to have. She was so happy.

Like many women, her miscarriage (it seems so wrong to even call it that at that stage), was unexpected and debilitating to her and her husband.

'Can you help us?' he asked—pleaded with us.

Anna didn't know he was contacting us. He didn't know what to do to support her.

I realised, in that moment, that our experience made us different. Special. Useful. It gave us a perspective that would never leave us but could help other people.

My heart broke for her. Her husband had reached out to Chris the day they had found out, asking what to do and how to support his wife. I spent hours thinking about what I could say to her, how I could use my experience to support her and I realised that there was so much I had learnt over the last nine months.

It was early days for them so, in the short term, none of what I had learnt would probably help her in the initial days.

When I first said goodbye to Violet, I devoured the online stories of others who had walked in my shoes, but I hated receiving direct advice from those I knew. I didn't want to be told that it wouldn't hurt this bad forever. I didn't want to know that eventually I would have weeks without crying and would be a functioning member of society again.

But I could still be a supporter. I just had to let her know I was there; she was not alone, and this situation completely and utterly sucked.

So, when I messaged Anna, I told her I was there for her to message anytime, I sent her love and strength during what I knew would be difficult days and nights. I didn't provide advice, but I did ask if she needed any practical suggestions or support with things such as urns, books about baby loss, recommendations to online groups and how to break the news to others.

Later, I could provide more specific practical advice.

I could let her know that there is no 'getting back to normal' or 'getting over it'. There is only a new normal.

In one of our messages, Anna apologised to me in case her loss brought up any emotions for me. I responded by telling her never to apologise for her loss and I also let her know that my sad feelings are always there. They haven't left and I haven't gotten over it—this is something I realised she didn't know yet. This inspired this chapter on everything I wish I knew but wouldn't have listened to if you had told me and most likely wouldn't have believed even if I listened.

To help write the chapter, I asked a group of other loss mums what some of the things were that they wish they had known before or during their loss.

Many of them said that they wish they had known how common baby loss is.

In Australia, the statistics show approximately one in four pregnancies will end in loss.

**Every day in Australia**
Six babies are stillborn.
Three babies die within the first twelve months of birth.
A miscarriage occurs every 3.5 minutes.

The reason the statistics around pregnancy loss are reassuring to those who have experienced it is because it helps you know you aren't alone. However, it is important to note that it doesn't change the fact it happened to you and certainly doesn't make the pain any easier to deal with. Knowing the statistics helps you understand that far more people have a story than you realise.

Prior to actually giving birth to their babies, many loss mums wished that they were more prepared.

Those who gave birth to their babies wish they knew not

to be so scared about what their baby would look like. Almost everyone I spoke to was nervous prior to giving birth about what condition their baby would be in and how they would look once they arrived. But to each person their baby was absolutely beautiful, and they felt nothing but love when they saw them.

A couple of people mentioned that they wished they were prepared for how long it would be between finding out that their baby's heartbeat had stopped and giving birth.

One mum, Kate, had it confirmed that her baby had passed away on a Sunday and then had to wait until the following Friday before she was induced.

This was something that also surprised me. I thought once we had decided, it would happen quickly. Our decision was made on a Thursday, and I wasn't induced until the following Thursday.

Once everyone had given birth, they mentioned wishing they were more prepared for the hormonal changes and response their body would have after giving birth.

They wish they knew that their milk would come in and even if they had taken the tablet to stop it, it would still feel incredibly painful.

Once a bit more time had passed for Anna, and she was in a place she was able to talk about her experience more freely, I shared with her some of the important lessons I have learnt.

I have learnt that it is okay to talk about my baby as much as I want to and that I eventually stopped caring about the responses and reactions of others.

In my experience, the more I speak about Violet the more people seem to accept her as a part of my life. Those who couldn't make eye contact in the initial days when I would discuss her are now just used to it.

I have learnt that including Violet as a member of my family and developing rituals where she is included is incredibly important to me. Also, having projects like this book and Violet's Gift has helped me in feeling connected with her and others.

I have learnt that there is a whole community of women out there who have also experienced losses. The loss mama community is supportive and non-judgmental. There is no shame, blame or awkward silences. I have learnt that speaking to other women who have a shared experience is incredibly helpful in healing.

I have learnt that although social media can be incredibly helpful, it is important to set some guidelines.

Spending too much time looking at other people's happy families and babies is not good for my mental health. I also have to remind myself that social media provides a glimpse of other people's highlight reels and wouldn't even tell one quarter of their story.

I have learnt that everyone's experience of loss is their own. Every story is uniquely different, and the way people learn, heal and grieve is entirely personal.

I have learnt that my feelings, responses and reactions to things will not always be the same. Some significant milestone days like Christmas may be challenging, whilst others might come and go without much fuss. I might be able to hear about someone's pregnancy without a second thought and others might leave me a blubbering mess.

I have learnt that people won't know how to respond to you, and you might need to explicitly tell them what you want and need. Most people in your life genuinely want to help and be there to support you but they don't know how. Sometimes a bit of explicit direction is all they need.

I have learnt that it is okay to be happy and celebrate life again. I realised that being happy doesn't mean I love or miss my baby any less. Her presence is in everything I do, and her existence has made me the person I am today.

During my research, the term 'microchimerism' is something I read about that really comforted me. During every pregnancy the mother and child exchange a small number of cells. This is called microchimerism. This means that every mother has a biological connection with every child created in her womb at a cellular level until she dies. No matter whether they are born, miscarried, stillborn, aborted or terminated for medical reasons.

I love the idea of this so much as I always feel like Violet is a part of me—in my cells, in my skin and in my blood. And I am a part of her too.

Our stories and lives will be interwoven forever.

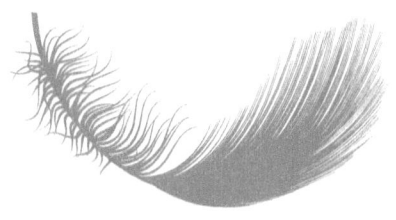

*I have learnt that it is okay to be happy and celebrate life again. I realised that being happy doesn't mean I love or miss my baby any less. Her presence is in everything I do, and her existence has made me the person I am today.*

## CHAPTER FOURTEEN
# Still a Mum

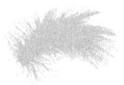

As I opened the card and read the message inside …

> Dear Mum, Happy Mother's Day! Thank you for all your love, and all that you do. I love you so much, you truly are the best Mum in the entire universe!

… I couldn't help but shed a tear. The card was signed 'love Baby Vi' but it was written by my husband. This isn't unusual when your child was only born a year earlier but most mums know that, sometime in the future, their little girl or boy will be signing their name themselves—or a wibbly wobbly version of their initials in crayon.

This isn't my reality.

Mother's Day can be a wonderful day for many women. A day of celebration, honour and love. But for those of us with children gone too soon, it can be a day of dread, sorrow and longing. We are mothers, but the world can sometimes forget, especially if we no longer have living children to carry and to hold.

Mother's Day was another milestone day that I really wasn't

looking forward to. It felt like another day where I would be reminded of the fact my daughter died.

Like most significant days for me, the thought of what it meant was actually more upsetting than the actual day.

On the Friday and Saturday before Mother's Day I received multiple flower deliveries from close family and a close friend. Our house felt so full of love as everywhere I looked were beautiful bright blooms.

I was gifted a candle and earrings 'from' Violet and spent the day being spoilt with all of my favourite foods and activities. My phone kept beeping with messages from friends wishing me a Happy Mother's Day.

I even received messages from people I wasn't that close to and hadn't spoken to in a while. Many of the messages were a simple 'Happy Mother's Day', some people acknowledged they didn't know if saying Happy Mother's Day was the right thing to say—but it was important that they felt I was acknowledged. Many other people also said how lucky Violet is to have such a strong and inspiring mum.

If you'd told me when Violet was born that I'd one day be able to enjoy this occasion, I would never have believed you, but it's amazing how the passing of time can shift your reactions.

To my surprise, my heart was bursting with love for the whole day. I felt so proud to be Violet's mum and to be celebrated for my role.

It wasn't until later in the day when I was scrolling through social media that I realised my reaction and the way that my loved ones showered me in love wasn't common.

In fact, many mothers who lose babies don't feel like they can celebrate Mother's Day, and aren't celebrated by the people around them.

As I scrolled through social media and read the comments of other parents whose children are no longer with them, it broke my heart to hear their heartbreak—those who dread the day and wish they could just sleep through it, those who feel invisible, mothers crying in secret.

When I returned to work the Monday after Mother's Day, I was also reminded that many people in my life don't know how to acknowledge my role as a mum, and whether I still see myself as one.

I began the day in a meeting with five other people—three mums and two dads. One of the dads asked if everyone had a good Mother's Day, then went on to specifically ask each mum if she was spoilt and the other father what he did for his wife. I waited for my turn to be questioned too, but it didn't come.

When he looked at me, instead of asking about my day, he suggested we begin the meeting. This person knew about my story and Violet but, I can only assume, they had no idea how to acknowledge or address my role as a mother. I wasn't upset or offended, but it did make me wonder about how I felt about my place in society too.

Having your motherhood ignored on a daily basis is painful and days like Mother's Day often only highlight it.

When I catch up with my friends and they all talk about babies and pregnancy, I listen but very rarely contribute unless asked or included. I know I am not alone in this. Because most of the time, although there are aspects of motherhood we can relate to, it is often awkward when we share them or add them into a conversation when you are talking about your living children.

There are many people who probably don't classify me as a mum. And it's true, there are many aspects of motherhood I can't relate to:

> I am a mum, but I have no idea how to change a nappy.
> I am a mum, but I have never gotten up in the night to a crying baby.
> I am a mum, but I have never purchased baby clothes for a child of my own.
> I am a mum, but I have never heard a little person call me mum.
> I am a mum, but I don't have a baby in my arms.

However, everyone says that once you become a mum, your world completely changes, and that is something I know to be true.

If you ask me when I think I became a mum, it wouldn't be as simple as the moment I held a positive pregnancy test or the moment I held our daughter in my arms. I remember when I was first pregnant, I used to say things like, *I can't wait until I'm a mum.* But now I've realised I already was one—as soon as I began thinking, dreaming and considering bringing a child into this world, my role changed forever.

One year before, I remember celebrating my own mum on Mother's Day discussing how I couldn't wait to be celebrated as a mum when our baby arrived. My view on motherhood has changed so much since then.

It's not as clean cut as you might think, not being a mum, conceiving and then becoming one instantly.

The definition of mother in the Merriam-Webster dictionary is a female parent. But upon reading countless pages and definitions, the meaning of a mother/mum is virtually endless. I even asked some of my friends and family what they thought defined someone as a mum and their responses were all different.

Here are some of their thoughts:

> A mum is someone who is there through thick and thin and loves you no matter what.

> Being a mum means that your baby is the first thing you think of when you wake up and the last thing you think of when you go to bed. Nothing else seems to matter much but them.

> Mums can look different and cross gender boundaries depending on individual situations. It may even come down to a maternal feeling towards others.

There are new mums, mums with multiple children, working

mums, single mums, step mums, adoptive mums, foster mums and mums who have lost babies and children. There are many people who are mums in their heart, but their bodies aren't cooperating.

I spoke to two friends who have experienced miscarriages, and one proudly refers to herself as a mother to her babies that she lost. Both of her babies have gender-neutral names as it was too early to find out their gender. She openly talks about them and she has dedicated part of her life to creating pregnancy loss resources in their honour.

My other friend, Ash, said she didn't really feel like a mum during or after her miscarriages. She told me in all honesty she didn't really ever feel like she had lost a baby. She said it felt more like she had lost the possibility of being a mum. The hardest part of that period of time was never knowing if she would have living children of her own and be a mum.

Two years later, once she held her son in her arms, she felt like a mum for the first time.

Another couple of my friends have stepchildren. When they met their partners, their partners both had children to previous people. Both of my friends find the title of mum or step mum incredibly tricky. They have been conscious of not pushing to be the kids' mum or replace their birth mum, but on the other hand, still treating the kids as their own.

They do their washing, cooking, cleaning, buy presents for their friends, remember all the important information and care for them as any mum would, but they don't get any of the recognition. It is something that they both have struggled with and continue to struggle with, even more so with the addition of their own children.

Through conversations, reading different perspectives and my own personal experiences it is clear to me that there is no set definition of a mum that fits everyone. It's incredibly complicated.

Before welcoming Violet, I thought it was as simple as: grow up, meet a boy, buy a house, get married and have a baby. I hadn't considered anything further than that. I hadn't thought about things like IVF, adoption, fostering and all of the other ways you can become a mum. The last year has been a crash course in what motherhood can look like, and why you should never judge a woman or her status as a mother by a child hanging off her hand—or the lack of one.

I can clearly remember the first time I was called a mum by someone else and how happy it made me feel to hear it. It was a couple of days before Violet was born, she was alive and moving around in my tummy, but I knew our time together was soon going to come to an end. I had reached out to a woman on social media who had also lost a baby under similar circumstances. Just before I went into hospital, she delivered a special giftbox to my house and on the card it read: *From one mama to another.*

I had heard many women and mothers before me explain the protective mother instinct you feel when you become a mum. As my beautiful baby grew in my tummy, I began to feel that instinct every time I placed a protective hand over my ever-growing belly.

I still remember the night Violet was born and we were moving from the birth suite to our room in the hospital. The well-meaning midwife asked if I wanted to cover Violet up as we transported her in her cot. I understand why she suggested it, but I remember feeling so proud of her, I couldn't possibly conceive the idea of covering her up. I also felt incredibly protective and was prepared to challenge anyone who dared make an insensitive comment about her in my presence.

After Violet was born, when the photographer came to take our family photos, it still made me so happy when he referred to me as 'Mum' and to Chris as 'Dad'—despite the toughest circumstances. I remember how proud I felt to be acknowledged as a mother. Up until those moments, I hadn't really referred to myself as that because I felt like I didn't quite deserve the title and felt like a bit of an imposter.

One day after Violet was born when I was questioning my role in motherhood, I even desperately googled the definition of a mother to see if it would make me feel better about giving myself the title.

But now I realise: I am a mother and I will be one forever.

Being a mum to me means having more love in my heart for another being than I could have possibly ever imagined. It means thinking of and considering my baby with every life decision. Being a mum means loving and caring for another for the rest of my life. Being Violet's mum is by far the greatest gift I have ever been given.

Motherhood has been the most amazing and most challenging role I have had to date. It has pushed me to tears more than once and has me questioning almost every decision and choice I make. It has made me feel incredibly proud and protective.

I love being a mum because it has given me perspective. Violet has truly helped me see what's important in life. She has taught me lessons in love, resilience, grief and loss and truly helped make me the person I am.

> I am a mum who loves my child with all my heart.
> I am a mum who is selfless and sacrificed my own wellbeing for the needs of my child.
> I am a mum who gave birth to a beautiful baby girl.
> I am a mum who kissed every inch of my baby and sang endless lullabies.
> I am a mum who read countless books to my baby.
> I am a mum who only wants the best for my child.
> I am a mum who will continue to parent and consider my baby in everything I do for the rest of my life.

I've also realised that, as a mother, it's important that I find ways to celebrate and commemorate our family and my role in it. It would be all too easy to side-step moments like Mother's Day and not take the time to acknowledge who I am and the special child Chris and I created.

This is why, to me, occasions like International Bereaved Mother's Day are important—a day that exists specifically for mums like me. Started by Carly Marie Dudley in Australia, International Bereaved Mother's Day takes place every year one week before traditional Mother's Day. It is a day for any parent who has lost a child, and, in particular, honours mothers who have experienced miscarriage, stillbirth, SIDS, or any type of pregnancy and infant loss.

Like many things, prior to having Violet, International Bereaved Mother's Day was something I had never heard of before. (There is also an International Bereaved Father's Day that takes place one week before the traditional Father's Day.)

I know these special occasions bring a lot of comfort to a lot of parents and make them feel less invisible. Perhaps, in years to come, I will celebrate them in a bigger way. But this year, it didn't feel quite right for me—my child still feels so alive in many ways, I can still feel her in my arms and remember, so vividly, the moment she joined us.

This year, I received a few messages from friends on International Bereaved Mother's Day and I was grateful for them. I was also happy the occasion shone a light on bereaved mothers and opened up conversations, but I specifically chose to celebrate traditional Mother's Day instead, rather than seeing my role as separate. Personally, we prefer to think of ourselves as parents—in the present.

Although right now we have no idea if we will be able to give Violet siblings, we are still hopeful and have had many discussions about how we will talk to them about Violet.

Our hopes for Violet's possible future siblings are that they will always know about their big sister and understand that she is an incredibly important part of our family. We have already spoken about so many elements of our family dynamic—

including our firstborn child. How we will choose their names to match Violet, talk about her all the time, have her photos on the walls and keep Violet's belongings in a special personalised wooden keepsake box to show them.

I can't wait until the day I can sit on the floor and share all of her special things with her brothers and/or sisters. I look forward to showing them her teddies and blowing bubbles with the bubble wands from her memorial.

I do spend time thinking about growing our family, even though nothing is guaranteed. There are books about grief you can buy for siblings whose older sister or brother has already passed away. It explains how someone came before them and helps them to understand. We also hope to be as honest as possible when we talk about what happened: your big sister was very sick, which is why she couldn't stay with us.

We want any of Violet's siblings to know that they are here because she helped them on the journey.

It's another reason I'm writing this story—so one day they'll have this book to read when they're older and understand how much we wanted Violet and them too. We want any future children to think of Violet as an angel watching over them. We hope that they find comfort in knowing she is always with us all and gives them courage in all they choose to achieve and do in life.

I know from my experiences with children that they actually understand and accept a lot of these more challenging concepts far better than adults do.

How many children do I have? I know it's a question I'll be

asked in the future, especially if I'm pregnant. *Is this your first pregnancy? Is this your first baby?* I suspect the truthful answer will make some people uncomfortable, but I also know I couldn't answer any other way than 'No, it's actually my second baby, my first was stillborn.'

I'm not saying that I'll never gloss over the truth—who wants to get into their medical history with a stranger in a supermarket queue? But, generally, I think that honesty is the best policy and will stop me from feeling like I'm dishonouring our eldest daughter.

In the future, if I have two more children and someone asks me how many kids I have, I know that it will forever be a challenging question—just like when people ask me now if I have any kids. In my heart and with my family and friends Violet will always be my eldest child and she will always be included. But just like if people ask if it's my first, it might depend on the person and the situation, because although Violet always deserves to be acknowledged, not everyone deserves to hear her story.

If you ever ask anyone how many kids they have and they share with you that one of their children was stillborn or miscarried, don't awkwardly move on. Sit in the uncomfortable and ask them the names of ALL their children. Ask them how old they are and when their stillborn baby was born.

My advice for how to support a bereaved friend on a day like Mother's Day is similar to my advice for any significant day:

- Acknowledge that this day may be painful or difficult for them: 'I know this may be a hard day. Please know I'm thinking of you.'

- Say their baby's name. I can't stress this enough. Hearing our babies' names said by other people is like magic.

- Acknowledge that they are a mother. Let them know you remember they are a mum even though their child is no longer alive.

- Send a Mother's Day card or message and include them in the celebrations.

Just because my baby isn't here doesn't mean I'm not a parent, I know I will continue to parent Violet every day. Just not in the way we had hoped or originally planned.

Whether or not I go on to have another child, I will always be a mother—whether my child is visible to the world or not. Despite what anyone else thinks, I am still a mum.

If you've lost a child, you are always a mum to me too.

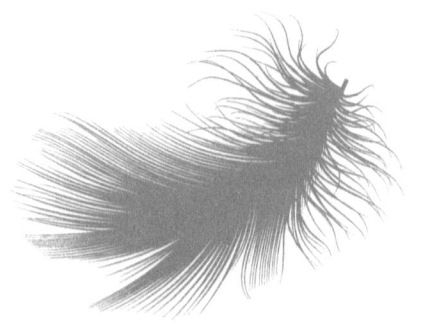

*Now I realise: I am a mother,
and I will be one forever.*

## CHAPTER FIFTEEN
# Through Dad's eyes

There's something intrinsically special about hearing your baby's heartbeat on the sonography scans—an innate, almost primitive moment in which nothing else matters, and you would do anything and everything to protect that.

So, what happens when you know that you can't protect it? What happens when your perfect little heartbeat is sick?

I remember the week between our last consultation with the genetics team, when it was decided that Violet's life couldn't be saved, and our admission to the hospital birthing suite. It was our last week together. It's strange to say that such an emotionally trying time can also be the most rewarding experience, but it's true: I became a dad for the first time.

During that final week with Violet in Meagan's belly, we made sure we relished every moment we had together as a family. We put headphones on Meagan's baby belly so that we could listen to music together and dance. (Violet wasn't the biggest fan of our music choices, but she did dance her little legs off to City and Colour's 'The Girl', which is fitting and will always hold a special place in my heart.)

We read all the picture books, and broke down and cried on each page. We watched all the kids movies, ate all the food, and just experienced life together as a family for the first time, in whatever way we could. That week was a rising crescendo of love and heartbreak leading up to the moment when baby Violet was born.

I'll save you the details of the birth, but it has to be mentioned that Meagan is the strongest, most resilient woman I know, and both Violet and I are extremely lucky to have her in our lives. The medication necessary to induce labour has a drastic, almost violent impact on the human body and Meagan, to her credit, was as stoic, strong and brave as ever.

Violet was born at 1.40am in the cold, dark hours of the winter morning. The room was silent. Seeing Meagan and Violet together broke me—my two girls together at last.

The nurses left us to be a family and understandably Meagan soon drifted off in a much-deserved rest as the medications took control.

I didn't sleep at all that night, I sat up next to Violet and just looked over her throughout the morning; as I write that, it sounds so poignant and beautiful, but in reality, I had a constant stream of tears and was a total mess.

It's hard to put into words how I was feeling at the time— was my heart broken? Or was my heart so full of love that it was overflowing? I'd like to think it was the latter, but it's probably a combination of the two.

We had no real expectation or understanding of each other in terms of our stay at the hospital. Our original discussions were centred around giving birth and going home the next day if all things were clear from a medical perspective. This was coming from a space in which we didn't want to be a burden and felt the need to 'do the right thing' by freeing up hospital resources.

Thankfully, our mind frame changed and we spent three love-filled, amazing days together over the weekend. Our families were able to come and visit, which was all the more special as they all became aunties and grandparents for the first time.

For me, my favourite memory of this time was simply laying on the couch, watching our football team with Violet laying on my chest (Violet is a keen North Melbourne supporter), feeling her weight on me. It was a beautiful way for us to connect and is something I will treasure forever.

I now wear a necklace with some of her ashes in it, so that I can continue to feel that weight and connection, and know that she's always with me, guiding me through my days.

It's so true when I say that she's always with me, always guiding me on my journeys. Because of Violet, I definitely pause more and take in the natural beauty of the world. I'll see stunning vistas of the sun rising in the morning, the sky awash with picturesque hues of red, purple and blue, and it instantly transports me back to my time with Violet, and I thank her for giving me that beautiful little reminder.

I'll see rainbows after a storm and it's the perfect metaphor for our journey. Violet is the last colour in the rainbow and she's definitely the beautiful glimmer of hope and love after a tumultuous stormy day.

Even the little things remind me of my daughter, for example the colour purple. It's such a rare colour to come across that when I spot it and have the opportunity, I go towards it and it reminds me that everything is okay.

Purple, especially violet, is symbolic of nothing but pure, unfiltered, unrelenting and unconditional love to me.

As I write this, it's Violet's first birthday in a few weeks and, no doubt, I've grown and adapted over the past twelve months.

I was interviewed and featured in a very special book, *Miles Apart: A heartfelt guide to surviving miscarriage, stillbirth and baby loss*—a beautifully touching exposition on the tragedy of infant loss authored by Annabel Bower.

This interview took place just four weeks post Violet entering the world and, reflecting back at my responses, my journey with grief has definitely evolved over the months that followed.

Yet, it must be said that some things have remained the same.

When I see a random dad with his little girls doing completely normal, almost trivial things like food shopping or walking their dogs, my heart sinks.

It isn't necessarily a bitter, jealous or even angry response that comes over me. It's a reminder of the feelings I felt when I was with Violet for the first time, holding her close. It takes me back to that space when we were together and everything was okay.

Even though it triggers some sadness, I also find myself happy for that random dad—that he is doing his best and all that he knows is that unrelenting and uncontrollable feeling of love.

Whilst this feeling remains the same to this day, some of my reactions have definitely changed. Looking back to the early weeks and months of my grief, I was definitely hurt, broken and a little bit lost in the world, which is totally understandable.

As Meagan also discovered, some people didn't really know what to say; some would offer their sympathies, share their 'happened to a friend' story, or offer up the classic 'at least' statements.

Something that really resonated with me at the time was feeling lost in the world and very much on the outer, or as 'the other'. There is a great tragedy in feeling like you don't belong; ultimately, we as humans want to fit in, and find our people.

Unfortunately for me, I was now in a super exclusive club that had the shittiest and most expensive entry fee of all—the Infant Loss Club.

Reflecting on these statements, I've learnt that I would've placed myself in this outer as a way to protect myself, and to simply survive. I've also learned that the majority of people—as honestly silly as some of the things they say are—come from a loving place and are merely trying their best to engage with you, and to make you feel like you're not alone.

This whole experience has given me a crash course on perspective. I've always liked to think that I'm relatively genuine and authentic in my interactions with others and I try my best to be a nice guy, but now I have a greater appreciation for the unknown, the behind-the-scenes of each and every person's life. I also have a greater appreciation and understanding that we all have our own baggage that we carry around with us each day, and that we need support, kindness and love to help each other.

When tragedy strikes, or life becomes that little bit harder, I'm much more aware of how people are feeling, what to say and how to act, and find myself being able to sit with people in their emotions and be there together.

I don't find myself having negative, angry or jealous moments anymore. The *Why me?* thoughts have left, and life, although completely different and totally unexpected, has regained some form of normality—if only a different and new sense of 'normal'.

Meagan, Violet and I are a family, and we grow each day with love as a family does. We talk about her all the time, we light her candle, we sing, we dance, we include her in everything we do, because she is our special little girl. Even more so, she makes us special too. She has given me the greatest gift of all; I'm her dad.

Truth be told, that first Father's Day was rough! It came not that long after Violet was with us, and whilst it was a beautiful reminder and a truly special day, my god … it hurt so much. She gifted me these adorable little socks and every time I wear them, she helps me take the steps through life. It's just one of many little reminders I get of her each and every day.

Moving forward, Violet has given us the greatest gift of all—an opportunity to grow our special family if we choose to explore this option.

The genetic testing undertaken on Violet was able to pinpoint and locate specific genetic issues that made her so sick. With targeted genetic IVF treatment and planning, there's a chance that we'll be able to have more kids.

I am literally blown away by modern science and advancements in medical technologies.

Whilst this is a book about Violet, there has to be a small section dedicated to Meagan.

Throughout this whole experience, she has grown into herself and become the very definition of a mother—loving, kind, unwavering with her support and oh so strong. She has been to hell and back, both physically and mentally, yet the stoicism and grace she carries herself with each and every day garners my undying love, respect and gratitude.

Throughout this whole process, she has endured many extremes; infinite invasive tests, constant unknowns and a never-ending series of needles and injections, on top of losing her firstborn child. She would be well within her rights to pack it all in and quit, and I can definitely understand how many marriages and relationships fail after such testing times, yet that's not Meagan. She became stronger, wiser and more aware of the world, she became Violet's Mum. And together, we live each day honouring our beautiful little girl and ensuring that her name is never forgotten.

If you're a dad who is unfortunate enough to find yourself in a similar situation, my advice is to feel the full force of your emotions. Ditch the male bravado, and really listen. Listen to your partner, listen to yourself and listen to your heart. Display your emotions. You're grieving. Say your baby's name, say it loud and proud.

There is a stereotypical view in contemporary society that the dad has to be the 'man of the house'—the strong, silent type. Sure, there are some merits to that idyllic way of life, however in situations like this, it serves zero purpose. Being silent just causes harm.

Talk to your partner. Talk about your beautiful little baby boy or baby girl. Talk about all the special moments you had together, however frail and fleeting they may have been.

Talk to your mates, make them comfortable talking about uncomfortable things—so that you can all grow and develop. Who knows, maybe in the future one of these mates will feel more comfortable talking about their own hardships.

There is no 'easy fix' or bandaid remedy for losing a child, it's something that changes your identity and that you carry with you forever. And yes, it is entirely confronting and brutally raw, but you owe it to your child. Be in touch with your emotions, show compassion, and love unconditionally.

So my final piece of advice is just that—love unconditionally, and grow together with your child, do everything you can to be the best version of yourself that you can possibly be, and do it all in honour of your baby.

*Display your emotions. You're grieving.
Say your baby's name, say it loud and proud.*

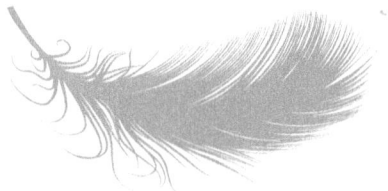

## CHAPTER SIXTEEN
# Never forgotten

When I look back on the moment I swallowed the pill that stopped my pregnancy hormones and began the process of ending my very wanted pregnancy, it feels like it happened to another person in another lifetime. I still don't know how I found the strength to do it or the courage to wake up the next week and face our new normal—as the parents of a stillborn baby.

When I think of all the significant milestones that Chris and I have experienced since then—Violet's due date and our first Christmas—I wonder how I got through those first few months. My heart breaks when I think about the pain we went through and how the closest thing Chris and I had to a date was attending a pregnancy/child loss support group.

But here we are—still standing, still living, still loving each other and our daughter.

Twelve months have passed, I can happily say that I haven't 'moved on' from losing Violet, but I have moved forward. I am no longer in the depths of my grief where I could barely function and my days of crying are fewer and farther between.

My biggest worry when I knew that Violet wasn't going to be staying with us 'physically' was that she would be forgotten and that the world would 'move on' and expect us to move on as well. Expecting people to move on from a monumental loss is, I have realised, incredibly unfair.

I now know that we will never 'get over' Violet and 'move on' because for as long as I am alive, I will continue to share her story and she will always be my firstborn baby and an incredibly important part of my family.

When I reflect on the last twelve months of my life and the stages, pages and chapters I have written, there are many parts of this book that are difficult to read as they remind me of much more challenging times and also because many parts no longer reflect how I feel. But there is a lot that is still relevant.

The first chapter is titled 'Uncertainty and Optimism' and, although I was uncertain and optimistic about something entirely different while pregnant with Violet, that is exactly how I feel as I wait and wonder if we will be able to give Violet siblings.

Hearing people say Violet's name is still music to my ears and makes me feel so happy. Having her acknowledged as my daughter and a part of my family is still as important as ever and, although the texts I receive from friends of rainbows and violet flowers don't arrive as often, when I get them they make my day (although I also understand that, for my friends and family, my grief can't always be at the front of their minds—they have to begin to move forward with their lives too).

On International Women's Day on 8 March, someone I had only recently met sent me a message saying: 'It's beautiful that you can share your truth and experience time and time again.

I don't know if you know it but when you talk about Violet your eyes just light up. I can feel your soul, honestly. You are rewriting the rules on grief and you are doing such a graceful service to those around you and how they might deal with their own grief.'

I hope that's what I'm doing—through my everyday conversations and through this book too. I want to let people know there is life after loss. It's not the same life and it's not always easy (I still struggle with birth announcements and maybe I always will), but you can carve out a new life, a new dream, and it's okay to want to.

You can also rebel against how you think you should react or need to react to moments and memories. I have adjusted my expectations of myself and don't feel overwhelming guilt if I don't attend things because I'm feeling flat or because I know it will be too difficult for me. Overall though I am enjoying my life again and Violet plays a big part in that as she is with me every day in every way.

On 19 July 2020 we celebrated Violet's first birthday.

In the lead-up to the day, I was full of a range of emotions but I was surprised to find sadness wasn't really one of them.

Three weeks earlier, I had injected myself with our first IVF hormone. To combat my fear of needles, I had kept Violet's urn close by—a symbol of the importance of family, and why we were starting this journey.

I felt happy to be celebrating the first year of our darling girl, and I felt optimistic and hopeful about IVF and giving Violet a sibling or siblings.

It wasn't until the night before her birthday that I started feeling a shadow creep in.

A year ago to the day, I was in the birthing suite at the hospital and had been through hours of emotional and physical pain. Every hour that passed I knew it was less time we would have together. I felt Violet move around for the last time in my belly without knowing I would never feel her move again.

I remembered what it felt like to go through labour unsure if my daughter would be born alive and if she was, knowing that she wouldn't be able to stay for long. I remembered the reactions of everyone in the room and how sad everyone seemed to be. Then I remembered that it was almost a year since the last time I held my daughter in my arms.

But I have to accept these memories are a part of me and are part of honouring our journey together.

Leading up to Violet's first birthday, I was unsure how I wanted to celebrate. Did we want to have a party, or would it be too sad? If we had a party, who would we invite? Were we supposed to buy birthday presents and then what would we do with them? These were just a handful of the questions on my mind.

In the end, the decision was taken away from us and we couldn't have a party even if we wanted to, because her birthday fell in the midst of the COVID-19 pandemic. Sadly, due to a change in the COVID-19 restrictions we were also no longer able to have the opening of the hospital room our fundraising had paid for.

However, thankfully, two weeks before Violet's special

day, I was able to visit the hospital and see the hospital room, complete with a beautiful wall mural of the beach with a violet sky and hidden violets in the water lapping the sand.

In the months leading up to Violet's birthday, I had been in regular contact with the staff at the hospital. As with most things related to Violet's Gift, I was so overwhelmed by the generosity of others. We had been in contact with a lady who fundraised Cuddle Cots in memory of her daughter and after hearing our story she had decided to assist us in purchasing one for Violet's room and then donated one in memory of Violet. So, the hospital was now receiving two new Cuddle Cots and portable bassinets—an amazing achievement.

When I was invited to visit the hospital to look at all the work we had done, I was anxious. I hadn't been to the room since the day I watched the funeral director take Violet with him. How would I walk in there again?

However, entering that space I felt so full of love and so proud. The couch, paint and carpet looked amazing and the Cuddle Cot was beautiful. It was everything I wish that we had had during our time together.

Over the weekend of Violet's birthday, our house filled up with flowers as we received delivery after delivery. A couple of people sent cards in the mail and all of our close friends and family sent messages on her actual birthday. People sent photos of candles that they had lit and told us they were thinking of her.

Due to COVID-19 restrictions, we couldn't visit anyone, and no one could visit us. My sister and parents had their own little party, purchased some of my favourite pregnancy foods (i.e. Violet's favourite foods!) and set the table with violet and rainbow tablecloths. We also received a couple of special deliveries on our doorstep.

For each of my friend's children, I always give them books when they are born and for their first birthday. During the day one of my friends, on behalf of a group of them, dropped off a gift bag full of beautiful books for Violet's first birthday to be donated to the hospital room.

We also received an incredibly unexpected package from the beautiful team at the hospital. They had been creating a scrapbook of the journey of Violet's Gift and what we were creating together. It had photos, poems and kind words from midwives and people I had never met whom Violet's story had reached and touched.

When we thanked them, they said it was the least they could do and they had more pages to add, including from the room opening whenever we may have it.

We decided to make a donation to a pregnancy loss charity in her memory and Chris wrote her a special picture book called *Where the Violets Always Grow*.

On Violet's birthday, Chris and I spent most of our day making an elaborate cake. We decided we wanted it to incorporate all the things that remind us of Violet—rainbows, the colour and butterflies.

After many hours on Pinterest and googling how to do different things, we created a five-layer rainbow cake with violet buttercream icing, rainbow sprinkles, fondant butterflies and a fondant rainbow.

We also learnt the lesson that for future birthdays the cake would be created the day before.

In one of my Pinterest searches I had come across beautiful cake toppers and purchased one that said *Violet is One*. It wasn't until the cake was created and we were getting ready to sing 'Happy Birthday' that I felt the cake topper was no longer appropriate. She wasn't one. She hadn't made it to one.

With tears in our eyes, Violet's urn next to us and our dogs at our feet we stood in our kitchen and sang 'Happy V Day', which is our rendition of 'Happy Birthday'.

I wrote to Violet that night in my diary and wished her a Happy V Day again. I thanked her for everything she had shown and taught me over the last twelve months and for choosing me to be her mum. I told her that I missed her and we thought of her every day and hoped she was proud of all we had done over the last twelve months.

The last twelve months since having Violet have been the biggest of my life and in so many ways I couldn't imagine that this is where I would be in life at thirty-one. This is not the story or journey I envisioned for myself. I didn't imagine having a stillborn daughter and I didn't imagine it would lead to a long road of genetic testing and IVF.

After months of waiting for test results and to see if IVF was an option for us, within one week we received the news that not only could we do IVF, but I had also collected the medications to begin our first cycle.

The reason I haven't wanted to wait to have another baby

before finishing this book is that I don't believe having another baby or being pregnant again is a happy ending. I am happy right now. Every time I speak of Violet my heart sings, she has turned the light up in every aspect of my life.

This is not the outcome that I ever wanted or would ever wish upon anyone, but it is my reality and instead of focusing on what I don't have, I choose to focus on everything I do have and everything Violet has helped me achieve.

Without Violet I wouldn't be the person I am today and I wouldn't have been able to do so many things. She has given me a strength and courage I didn't know existed.

I wouldn't have been able to help make changes to hospital policies, I wouldn't have been able to help others share their stories and I wouldn't have been able to make a difference to others who are also faced with the unimaginable through Violet's Gift.

As I come to the end of this book and think about sending it out into the world, I feel mixed emotions.

I feel sad that something I have worked so long on is finished.

Over the last twelve months this book has often felt like my main connection to Violet, as mentioned previously it has been an incredibly important part of my healing journey and it feels strange to be coming to a close. However, I also feel ready to move forward to the next stage of my life with Violet by my side.

There is a small part of me that is worried about how our

story will be received once it is out in the world in this way and I know that whenever you put yourself out there and share so deeply you are opening yourself up to the opinions of others. I also know though that every person our story helps to feel less alone and every person it helps to understand the complexities of pregnancy loss will more than make up for a negative comment or unkind opinion.

In general, I no longer worry about the reactions of others in my day-to-day life and I discuss Violet and remember her in a way that feels right to me. I've found that some people still react better than others and there are some people who definitely think I should be over it by now, but time has helped me not to care too much about other people's reactions.

When I started my new job, one well-meaning friend said, 'What a great opportunity where no one has to know your story, and you can start fresh.' I couldn't think of anything worse! I don't want to delete my past, but I do want to choose how and when to share it.

Through conversations with a close friend, I decided to make a video introducing myself where I would share a bit of my life and experiences personally and professionally. In the video I spoke about Chris and my dogs and told the staff about Violet:

> 'I have one daughter, Violet, who was stillborn in July last year. I am not telling you this to upset anyone or make anyone uncomfortable, I am telling you as being a married woman in my thirties one of the first questions I am asked is if I have any

children and I definitely do. Violet is my daughter and it is important to me to share that with you and ensure she is always acknowledged.'

By reading this book, you are acknowledging my daughter, so thank you for learning from her existence.

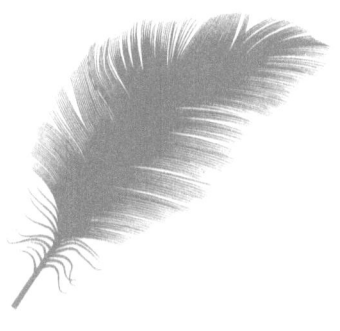

*Hug the people you love.
Look forward.
Accept that grief doesn't have to defeat you.
And always have hope, even in your darkest moments.*

*In sharing our story, I hope that Violet's life can become a gift to you too.
She never took a breath, but she will never be forgotten.*

BONUS CHAPTER
# Violet's impact

Violet will always have an impact on my life and an imprint on my heart, but what has surprised me since her birth and since I've started sharing our story more publicly, is the number of people who also say she's had an impact on their life too. Some of these people are obvious—my family, Chris's family and our close friends who lived our grief with us—but Violet has also touched people who we barely know, and that is part of her amazing legacy.

For this book, I asked some of these people to share what Violet's short life has meant to them, in their own words.

## JULIA, VIOLET'S AUNTY

When I held Violet in my arms the day after she was born, I felt such a powerful sense of all-encompassing love. That memory gives me great comfort, especially on days when I feel sadness about what happened.

Violet's life has, and does, make me think a lot about baby loss and the struggles so many people go through—the traumas they've experienced that we don't even know about.

Violet's life has made me much more mindful of this and the impact that asking a simple question like *Do you have kids?* can have on someone who has experienced loss or is undergoing IVF treatment.

I don't have any children of my own, but I feel so much love for my niece and I treasure being her aunty. Violet has reminded me of the power of love. I am an aunty because of her.

## LAURA, FRIEND OF MEAGAN AND CHRIS

I have known Meagan basically my whole life. Our friendship has become more like a sisterhood, which I'd like to think makes me one of Violet's honorary aunties.

When Meagan and Chris told me they were pregnant, whilst they were elated, it was always clouded with uncertainty. As a friend, my heart was full of excitement for them becoming parents. However, as a mother myself, the possible outcome made my heart heavy.

While I never got to meet Violet, she has taught me so much and, as clichéd as it sounds, it begins with a simple fact: life really is so precious.

I know how much Meagan and Chris cherished every moment they had with Violet. Now, this path has led them to honouring Violet's legacy—using their pain to help other families.

Violet might not have been with us earthside for very long but, my gosh, her parents have and are continuing to show their love for her.

## ROBIN, VIOLET'S GRANDPA

My wife and I have experienced loss through miscarriage but losing Violet has made me more aware of those around me who have gone through stillbirth or the loss of a child, and what they are experiencing.

Becoming a grandfather for the first time, but being unable to enjoy time with Violet and watch her grow, has been very upsetting. When other people share photographs of their grandchildren with me and tell me about their experiences, I'm sad and my heart hurts as I am unable to do the same.

I'll never forget the little girl I held who made me a grandpa. The little girl who will always be an important part of our family.

## AMANDA, VIOLET'S GRANDMOTHER

After raising three healthy, bonnie babies myself and watching them grow into successful adults, the grief and sadness I feel for my son and daughter over the loss of Violet is inconsolable. Babies aren't supposed to die. Parents spend their lives trying to protect their children but I could do nothing to stop this. I feel so helpless and my heart aches for their pain and loss.

I can still see Violet's dear little face the day I met and cuddled my granddaughter. I remember her long fingers, her toes and her smell, and I treasure that brief moment in time.

My son and daughter have tremendous strength, commitment and love. In writing this book, if it helps others in any way, it is a positive outcome. Love is the greatest healer.

I am Violet's grandmother and, for that, I am most grateful.

## SILVIA, FRIEND OF MEAGAN AND CHRIS

I am one of Violet's mum's best friends (a pseudo aunty!). Blessed with two beautiful kids.

I was not only heartbroken for my friend after the loss of their beautiful baby girl, but I felt personally robbed of our shared experiences.

I couldn't help thinking of all of the things we would miss out on doing together—being pregnant, playdates, sharing bad sleep stories and all the funny things our kids have said and done. This thought makes me sad, but all the big things my friends have accomplished in the past year makes me very proud of them too.

Violet has taught me gratitude for the little things in life. Once Violet's mumma said she never got to point out birds and flowers to Violet, and now I always to do that for my kids—and think of Violet when I do.

## EMILY, VIOLET'S AUNTY

I'll never forget the day I met my niece, Violet. I didn't know what to expect and I didn't want to say or do the wrong thing. But, my nerves were pushed aside as soon as I saw her—the most beautiful baby I had ever seen.

Perfectly formed, she was like a doll with her smooth skin and little button nose. I think about her every day and I'm so grateful for the time I had with her at the hospital where I was able to hold her, and see her parents and other family members form a special bond with her in their own ways.

The most prominent feelings that emerge when I think about Violet are naturally those associated with loss—all the milestones and the minutia of every day that she'll never get to experience with the rest of us.

However, with the heartache also comes hope and opportunities for reflection. I'm touched by the way Violet has connected so many people and opened up an important dialogue around loss. Violet's lasting legacy is one that promotes healing and that is something I'm so proud of.

## CAITLIN, FRIEND OF MEAGAN AND CHRIS

When Meagan asked if I would like to write some words on Violet's life and her impact on me, I kept coming back to the last two stanzas of a poem I recently came across called 'The Weighing' by Jane Hirshfield: *So few grains of happiness measured against all the dark and still the scales balance. The world asks of us only the strength we have and we give it. Then it asks more, and we give it.*

Violet is one of those grains of happiness and Meagan and Chris are a shining example of the unknown depths of strength that are within us.

I am about to become a first-time aunty and Violet's life is a reminder to me of the remarkable constellation of atoms that we are all made of and to constantly strive to live that gift with kindness and love.


## LAUREN, VIOLET'S AUNTY

I was so excited when I found out I was going to be an aunty for the first time. When things became uncertain it was really challenging for me as I didn't know how to be there for my sister. My heart broke when I found out things weren't going to be as we had all hoped.

I was scared to meet Violet at the hospital as I wasn't sure what she would look like, but that fear quickly disappeared once I saw her and got to hold her in my arms.

Violet made me an aunty and taught me what's important in life. She has made me more aware of pregnancy loss and how common it is. She has also helped me be more supportive of those that may struggle with fertility.

## DAWN, VIOLET'S GREAT NAN

It has been tough to watch the heartache that has affected my family—and my own heart—and not be able to do anything to help anyone, but it has brought lessons too.

In the past year, I have learnt to always stop and listen when people want to talk and never just say 'I know', because you don't really know until the same has happened to you. I know this now, through personal experience, from the people who have said the same to me.

Until you have to watch your own daughter grieving over her daughter's grief and the loss of her granddaughter, you can't imagine how that feels.

Violet was so wanted and loved by so many, and all of our hearts are broken in so many ways.

The short time Violet was here she was loved so much and always will be.

## LISA, FRIEND OF MEAGAN AND CHRIS

When I heard that Meagan and Chris had lost Violet, I was actually shocked at the level of my own grief and the depth of my emotions. I understood their loss from a logical perspective —this was a desperately wanted pregnancy and a much-loved baby—but I had no comprehension of the sense of loss that I could feel for someone else.

I am going to become a first-time nana later this year and

Violet has been in my thoughts so much during the pregnancy. I am grieving for the milestones that I know Meagan and Chris will never get to experience with Violet.

The biggest impact Violet has had on my life is an understanding that we have limited moments, regardless of how long we live.

In Violet's honour, I promise to always give the hugs, celebrate the small things and tell those close that I love them. I will look out the window and take a moment to appreciate the sun, the trees and the birds every day.

For me, Meagan and Chris have redefined strength, grace and humility—Violet chose her mum and dad well. I will be forever grateful to them for sharing their family's story with us all.

Violet is a little girl I never met but I talk about her, I talk to her and I will celebrate her life.

## LYNDA, VIOLET'S GREAT AUNTY

Twenty-five years ago when I married my husband, Meagan was our beautiful flower girl. I never thought that we'd be living through this experience together now.

Violet has been such a beautiful gift to our lives. Although she was only here for a short time, she has made a big impact on my life and my family's. She will always be remembered because every time I see a rainbow I think of her.

Violet has taught me that life is very precious and short, be happy and smile as often as you can, try and remember the good in life as hard as that can be at times.

## ERIN, FRIEND OF MEAGAN AND CHRIS

Violet's birth changed my perspective. After going through personal issues, her arrival allowed me to see outside of myself and begin to recover.

Although I knew how strong her mum was, I was and I am still amazed by her strength since then.

Thank you, Violet, for teaching me an important lesson: life is so unexpected and we should seize every opportunity.

## GAIL, VIOLET'S GREAT AUNTY

Violet's birth impacted my life greatly, because my heart broke for my niece and her husband, Chris. Although our circumstances are very different, I also know the pain of losing a child is indescribable.

I am the mum of three adult children, Abbey, 21, Seamus, 19, and our firstborn daughter, Cate—our angel in heaven who would be 23 years old this year.

Violet's birth brought many emotions to the surface, which I thought I had dealt with—but hadn't!

Years ago, I kept Cate's loss to myself in the hope I didn't upset others or make them uncomfortable, but Violet has taught me that talking openly about stillbirth brings awareness and understanding.

Violet's life brought me the strength that I searched for 23 years ago—the courage to talk about stillbirth with no stigma.

Thank you, sweet Violet, for that.

## AMELIA, COLLABORATOR ON THE FUNDRAISER VIOLET'S GIFT

Meagan and Chris reached out to me in November of 2019 in regard to collaborating on a special project, Violet's Gift. My company, Tilda & Moo, sells handmade bibs and other items. I've had the pleasure of creating beautiful baby products to help raise money for the Violet's Gift fundraiser—a campaign that holds a special place in my heart.

My partner and I have been lucky in that we personally haven't experienced the tragedy of losing a baby, however I have tried to support friends and family during their tragic experiences and be there for them in the best way that I can.

Both of our girls were born at the hospital that received a Cuddle Cot thanks to Violet's Gift fundraising. It brings me comfort to know that, if someone I love ever experiences a loss at this hospital, Violet's Gift is there to support families through tragic times.

## BROOKE, FRIEND OF MEAGAN AND CHRIS

Throughout Meagan's pregnancy with Violet, I tried to be a supportive a friend. After going through two years of trying to conceive and two miscarriages myself, I felt like I had some small level of understanding.

During this time, I also fell pregnant and was due only eight weeks after Violet's due date. Violet gave me the gift of a love-filled pregnancy because, from the moment I found out that there was a doubt over her ability to physically survive in this world, I stopped focusing on any of the negative things that come along with pregnancy and experienced extreme gratitude.

To me, Violet is my beautiful friends Meagan and Chris's angel baby. She is the best friend that my daughter, Evie, never got to meet and a reminder to me, as a parent, just how lucky I am to be able to hold my babies in my arms as well as in my heart.

## AMY, EDITOR OF THE BOOK, STILL A MUM

I mentor a lot of writers who want to share their life experiences in a book, article or podcast, but none have touched me as much as Violet's story. I read and edited each chapter of this book as Meagan wrote it. Unbeknownst to her, I was pregnant with our third child at the time (a pregnancy my husband and I were keeping on the down-low!).

When Meagan heard that I'd given birth, she actually emailed to apologise in case reading about her loss was upsetting during my pregnancy. She couldn't have been more wrong!

Reading about Violet's life as I grew a child of my own was a gift. It gave me gratitude, hope and resilience, especially during challenging parts of my labour. As I walked into the hospital to give birth, I thought about Violet—a little girl I've only ever met in a memoir—and knew that I was going to be okay. If Meagan had the strength to welcome her baby daughter, I knew that I could find the strength to do the same.

Some stories stick with you forever and this is one of them. I'm so thankful I could be part of this project, to ensure that Violet's short but impactful life is never forgotten and will go on to touch people across the world.

## MEAGAN, VIOLET'S MUM

I am the lucky person who gets to call myself Violet's mum.

Violet has impacted my life in more ways than I could ever imagine. Everyone says that becoming a mum changes you and they couldn't be more right. I feel so lucky and forever thankful that Violet chose me to be her mum.

Violet has helped me truly understand what is important in life, she has helped me understand what my priorities are and to not sweat the small stuff. Violet has helped me realise life is truly what we make of it.

I spent most of my twenties reading books about happiness and how to live my best life, but it wasn't until I had Violet that

I truly understood the messages.

I would never wish my experience or loss upon anyone, but I do wish that they were able to experience the lessons and perspective I have received along the way.

Another gift Violet has given me is the ability to sit with people in their moments of sadness, loss or grief. I no longer feel uncomfortable or worry about saying the wrong thing, I am just able to be there.

Violet has shown me how strong and resilient I am and given me a knowledge that no matter what life throws at me, I will be okay. Violet taught me how to look after myself and be passionate about what I believe in.

I love talking about Violet and sharing her story. The impact she has had upon the world constantly astounds me.

I know that Violet is here with me always and I feel incredibly comforted by that knowledge.

# Pregnancy loss organisations and resources

There are many incredible organisations and supports available for those who have experienced the loss of a baby. These are also a great resource for anyone supporting someone through pregnancy loss.

## ORGANISATIONS

**Sands Australia**
A not-for-profit for bereaved parents following pregnancy loss. Sands provides a 24/7 support line people can call, support groups, and events.
24/7 Bereavement Support Line: 1300 308 307
sands.org.au

**Bears of Hope**
Support for families who have experienced the loss of a baby. They provide resources and ways you can honour your baby.
Grief Support: 1300 11 4673
bearsofhope.org.au

**Red Nose Grief and Loss**
Providing specialised bereavement support for anyone affected

by the death of a baby or young child. Red Nose has a 24/7 support line, information on safe sleeping and contribute millions to research into the possible causes and preventions of stillbirth.

Red Nose Grief and Loss 24/7 support line: 1300 308 307

rednosegriefandloss.org.au

**The Pink Elephants Support Network**

A suite of emotional support resources to support and nurture as people navigate their miscarriages and fertility journeys.

www.pinkelephants.org.au

**Heartfelt**

A volunteer organisation of professional photographers dedicated to giving the gift of photographic memories to families who have experienced stillbirth or have children with serious or life-threatening illness.

Australia: 1800 583 768

New Zealand: 0800 583 768

heartfelt.org.au

# RESOURCES

**Heart Space book**
A grief workbook for women after the loss of a child or pregnancy.
heartspacebook.com

**Aila and Lior pregnancy loss personal declarations**
Support and healing words for mamas of pregnancy loss and baby loss through personal declaration cards and a healing-after-loss handbook.
ailaandlior.com

**Born to Fly by Tamara J. Whittaker**
A delicate picture book providing comfort and hope after pregnancy, baby and child loss.
tamaraj.com.au

**'You Could Have Been' by Annie-M**
A children's picture book for bereaved parents to read to their child who died, or didn't survive a pregnancy. It's filled with a parent's wonder of who their child could have been if they'd had the chance to grow up. The book is written to the child, so a parent can talk to them about their lost hopes and dreams, but most importantly, their love.
babylossproject.com/book/about-the-book

**Harpermartin baby loss journals**
A baby book for a baby who is forever in your heart.
harpermartin.com.au/baby-loss-journals

**Keepsakes by Nicoleta**
Jewellery and memorial keepsakes made with ashes, locks of hair and breastmilk.
keepsakesbynicoleta.com.au

**The Porcelain Urn Company**
A lasting way to remember a loved one is to have their ashes placed inside an exquisitely handcrafted porcelain cremation urn.
theporcelainurncompany.com.au

# Acknowledgements

It is with great appreciation that I give thanks to the special people who helped make *Still A Mum* a reality. This book is here because of the love and support of so many.

To Zoe, Sabine and Martine for helping us create the hospital room for bereaved parents and making our Violet's Gift fundraiser bigger and better than we could have imagined.

To Rebecca for walking us through each step of our pregnancy, helping us understand what each test meant and for reassuring me at times when I doubted everything.

This book could not have been written without my incredible writing mentor and editor, Amy. Thank you for believing in me and for trusting that people would want to read about Violet and our story. I appreciate your dedication in helping to bring my book to life.

To Natasha, for your expert guidance and making the process of publishing a book enjoyable. I am thankful for every conversation, suggestion and tweak you have made. My gratitude to the rest of the team at the kind press too.

A special thank you to those who shared their stories and experiences so generously with me; the other loss mamas I've laughed with, cried with and exchanged many late-night messages with.

To those who contributed to our bonus chapter and shared the impact Violet's short life has had upon them. The people who continue to talk about Violet, say her name, remember her and acknowledge her, thank you.

To every single friend, family member and colleague who has reached out and supported us. We are lucky in that there are too many of you to individually name, but our hope is that you know who you are. We have felt the kindness of every act. You have no idea how much you have helped us.

A special thank you to my mum, Deb, for allowing me to interview her for this book and for being my rock throughout every stage of the journey

To my husband, my biggest supporter, my best friend and Violet's dad, Chris. I could not have gotten through any of this without you. I am so thankful every day for your love, support and belief in me. You are the best dad in the world. We are so lucky to have you.

Lastly, thank you, Violet, for choosing me to be your mum. I am so proud and grateful that you came into my life even if you couldn't physically stay; you are with me always.

# About the author

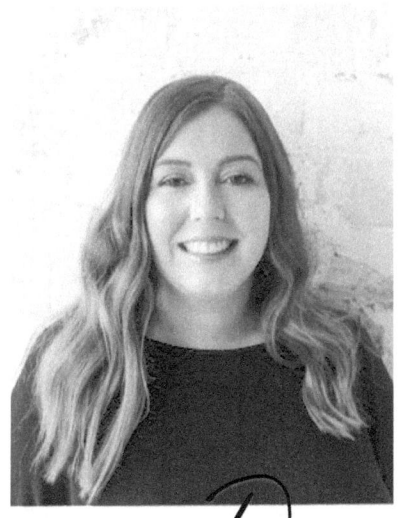

*Meagan Donaldson*

Meagan Donaldson works in education and is a writer. What's more, is that she is the founder of the fundraiser Violet's Gift. Which, in less than two months, raised over $16,000 to create a room in the hospital where her daughter Violet was born to support grieving parents after delivering a stillborn baby.

Meagan has spoken openly about her experiences of pregnancy loss and has collaborated with the hospital where her daughter was born to not only create the room but to change hospital processes.

www.meagandonaldson.com.au
Facebook: www.facebook.com/violetsgift
Instagram: @violets_gift

www.ingramcontent.com/pod-product-compliance
Lightning Source LLC
Chambersburg PA
CBHW022050290426
44109CB00014B/1041